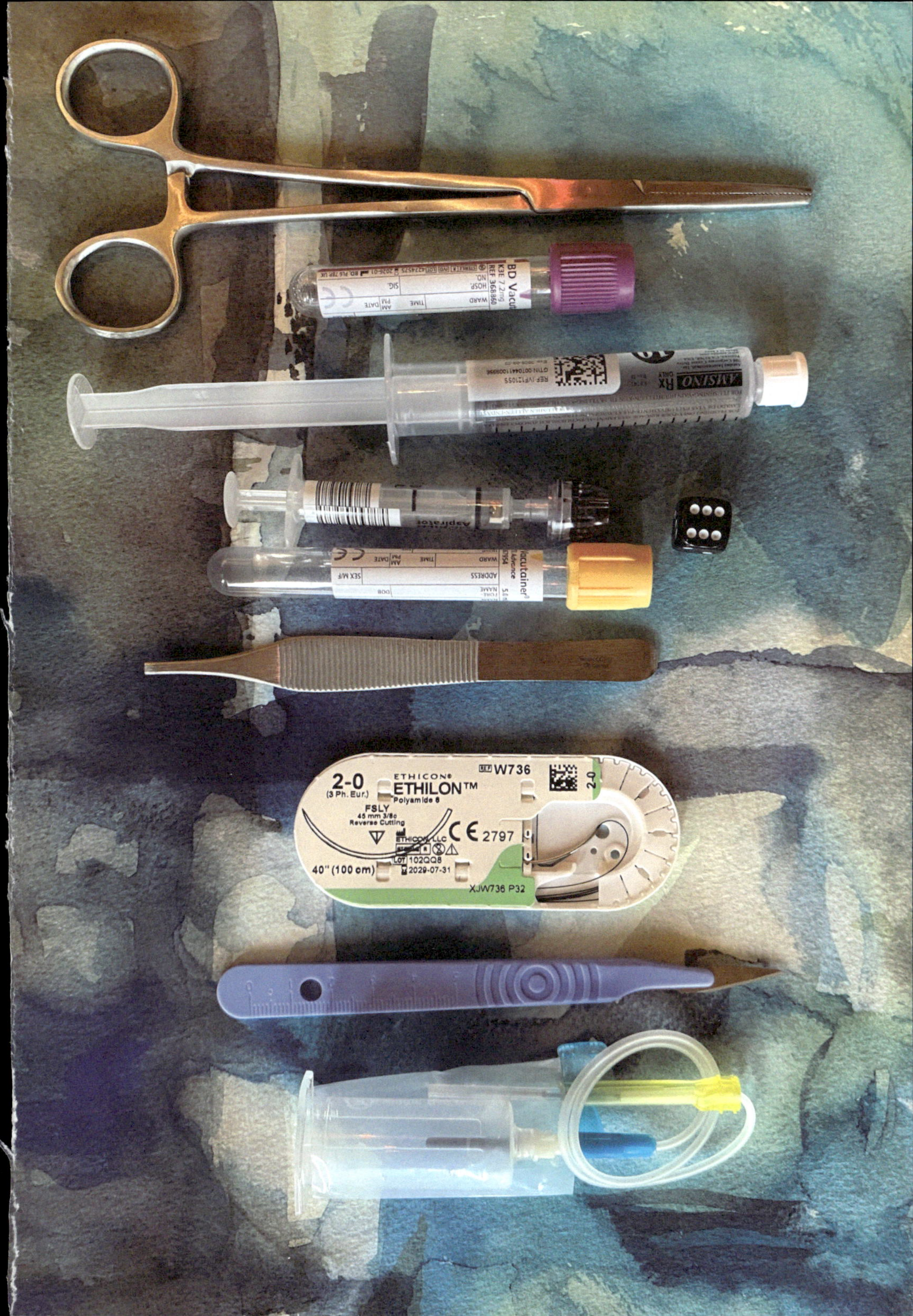
2-0
(3 Ph. Eur.)
ETHICON®
ETHILON™
Polyamide 6
W736
FSLY
45 mm 3/8c
Reverse Cutting
2797
ETHICON LLC
102QQ8
2029-07-31
40" (100 cm)
XJW736 P32

# BELLY
# FULL

ALSO BY HEIDI EDMUNDSON

*Darkness in the City of Light*

# BELLY FULL

Dr Heidi Edmundson

*Constellations Press*

First published in 2025
by Constellations Press

Typeset by Constellations Press
Printed and bound in the UK through Xpedient Book Print



A CIP record for this book is available from the British Library

ISBN 978-1-917000-07-9
e-ISBN 978-1-917000-13-0

*To my mother, Valerie Edmundson,*
*and my sister, Sarah Edmundson,*
*thank you*

# Prologue

This is a story about many things, including food, friendship, joy, sadness, dancing, despair, and my work as an Emergency Medicine consultant for the NHS. It's also a story about shame and fear, my shame and fear, that I carried around with me, hidden deep inside. I lived my life pretending to be the sort of person who did not have those kinds of feelings. They were my secret.

I rarely thought about them, but I always knew that they were there. I felt their presence like a fault line running through me. But most of the time, I managed to ignore them. Sometimes, now, I wonder if that is what the problem was. They got tired of being ignored and decided to make themselves visible. And when they decided to make themselves visible, let's just say, they made themselves very visible. So visible that, in the end, not even I, despite my best efforts, could continue to ignore them.

## January 2022: Be Careful What You Wish For

'We've really been left holding the fag end of the pandemic,' I said, as I reached for another tahini cookie. They were surprisingly moreish. One of the junior doctors had brought them in from a bakery in Hampstead. She had told herself that, as they contained tahini, they might be some kind of health food.

It was the beginning of January and I suspect that she, like a large proportion of the population, was on a diet. Of course, we don't call it 'being on a diet' anymore. It's not the eighties. We call it 'being a bit healthier.'

January is full of people being healthier. That morning, I had already discovered two people doing Dry January. One said he felt great. The other gave a grunt and muttered something about it only being a month. A very long month, though. Time, sometimes, is not equal. The thirty-one days of January are longer than the thirty-one days of other months.

That's why I am against the manufactured deprivations of Dry January and Veganuary. The month is hard enough as it is. Do what you can to get through it. I had reached a stage in life where I no longer believed in denial. I often joked that I was going to rename March as Starch and eat only carbohydrates.

However, in January 2022, I was definitely looking bigger; fat, to be honest. I couldn't fit into most of my clothes. At least, I suspected that I couldn't. I was instinctively avoiding any trousers with waistbands and zips. I found myself only wearing items made of jersey — stretchy, pull-on things — and even they were getting tight. It is a worry when even your comfortable clothes start feeling uncomfortable.

That New Year's Eve, I had struggled to find anything to wear, so I had decided that I, too, would need to 'be a bit healthier'. I was pragmatic. I had reached that age: the big M. It's great that we now all discuss the menopausal years openly. But it is also terrifying. It seems that anything can happen, overnight, in some cases. I only had few of the long list of symptoms, so I supposed that I was lucky. My burden appeared to be the menopause belly, and now I was ready to address it.

I didn't expect miracles. I wasn't expecting to be teenager-skinny; I had never been teenager-skinny, even when I was a teenager. I just wanted to be able to fit into my old clothes. As long as I can wear party clothes by next Christmas, I will be happy, I told myself.

But I allowed myself another half of a tahini cookie. People had started to do that thing where they halved the biscuits. Then they had another half when they had finished the first. Somehow, it seems less that way. Dieting is the one area where people hope that the total is less than the sum of all the parts. So, I had another half a cookie. It was Sunday morning, and I was at work. Sometimes you just have to do what you can to get through things.

'Yes,' I repeated. 'We have definitely been left with the fag end of the pandemic. Predictably.'

Everyone laughed.

Emergency Medicine is frequently left with the fag end of things. It seemed inevitable that when it was our turn to get hit heavily with COVID, no-one else was interested. At the start of 2022, no-one cared about COVID anymore; it was just a nuisance. Long gone were the sunny days of the first wave when the world was turned upside-down and we in the NHS were heroes. We were now well and truly in the new normal, which was very similar to the old normal, except a bit worse.

All the old NHS problems, which, for a brief time, seemed to have disappeared, were back with a vengeance: overcrowding, bed-blocking, treating people in the corridor. Of course, the cynics had said that they would never be resolved, and the cynics appeared to have been right.

Thankfully, due to the vaccine, treatments and successive waves, COVID was no longer the same as it had been at the beginning. Fewer people required admission, but large numbers of people were still coming in, crowding into the department with everyone else. And, like many others, they ended up stuck there. We had too many patients and too few beds, not to mention not enough staff. Worse, there was no end in sight. We were all exhausted and felt that we had no choice but to go on being exhausted or leave.

'COVID's like the Vietnam War,' I continued. 'We were clapped and cheered at the beginning but now, because we didn't win, everyone hates us.'

'You should write a book about it,' someone suggested.

'What, a big medical blockbuster, like Adam Kay or Rachel Clarke?' I asked. 'Then,' I added dreamily, 'I might make lots of money and not have to come in here anymore at the weekend.'

As it happened, I had already written one book and was working on my second. I wasn't writing them to make money; I knew that very few people make money from writing books. In any case, they were novels and had absolutely nothing to do with medicine. I wrote them partly to escape from my job as an Emergency Medicine consultant. I didn't know if I could bear writing about work after working all day — or, as I generally wrote first thing in the morning, before going into work all day.

The reason people write books is that they have a story to tell, but I didn't think I had the head space for this. Also, although I had undoubtedly lots of material after working as a doctor for nearly thirty years, I couldn't think of a way to bring it all together. I had no narrative hook on which to hang a story. I really should have remembered that old saying, 'be careful what you wish for.'

## Why I Became a Doctor

In April 2023, I was interviewed for a podcast and asked why had I become a doctor. Or maybe I wasn't; that's just how I remember it, and, let's face it, memory is an unreliable thing. Maybe I was asked how I ended up in the NHS, which is a slightly different question. But here is the story.

I was very young, pre-school probably. I was standing in our living room, and I was wearing one of those nurse's outfits that people frequently bought for little girls in the seventies. I was showing my grandmother; she might actually have bought it for me. I am really not sure of that, though. It's one of those occasions where I'm conscious that my mind is straying round the edges of a recollection and trying to create a story.

'When I grow up, I'm going to be a nurse,' I said.

'Oh no,' said my grandmother, 'don't be a nurse.'

My grandmother had been a nurse herself, leaving Ireland to train in Manchester. After Manchester, she had worked in Derby, met my grandfather, had my mother, been evacuated to Blackpool in the war, gone back home to Belfast, been evacuated to Bangor, and never nursed again.

'No,' she said, 'don't be a nurse, be a doctor, it's much better.'

Or maybe she said nicer.

Her rationale for it being better/nicer was that the doctors got very well looked after. They had their breakfast brought to them in the doctors' home, had their clothes laundered and their shoes cleaned.

My grandmother told me that her first job as a nurse was working in the respiratory wards. There she had to wash out the phlegm from the sputum pots and it 'turned her stomach.' She finished up by saying, 'Little girls can be doctors now, too.'

So, at some point in the early seventies, dressed as a nurse, I announced that I was going to be a doctor when I grew up, and that was that.

Once I'd said it, the idea pretty much stuck: all the way through primary school and then all the way through grammar school. I didn't really think too much about it. It just became what I was to become. I never thought about whether I would be good at it or if I would enjoy it. I never wondered if I would be temperamentally suited to it or if it would play to my strengths.

I've had conversations with many doctors about what we might have done instead of medicine. Or, to be more precise, what we *wish* we had done. I always choose something creative. My mind was much more creative than it was scientific. Sometimes I regret not having followed this path.

But, then again, who's to say I would have been any happier working in the arts or anything else? One huge advantage of medicine was job security. As a child of Thatcher's Britain, with a father who had been unemployed for a few years, I had a terror of not working.

Even when I went to medical school, I didn't think about it being a means to an end, the end being becoming a doctor. To me, medical school was all about becoming independent, having adventures, falling in love, and having fun. The studying was a necessary evil in order to justify being there.

It was only in the final year that the thought that I was to become a doctor began to creep up on me. I started to feel a little nervous. What stopped me feeling *extremely* nervous was that I had to pass my finals first, and that occupied the anxious part of my brain. When I did pass my finals at the end of June, there was very little time to be nervous, as I started working as a doctor at the beginning of August.

As it happened, being a junior doctor was not nearly as awful as I had feared. I settled into the job, and the job, as it was then, quite suited me. Back in those days, we were still working in a strong, team-based system. And being in a team very much matched my personality.

This way of working had both its positives and its flaws, with the biggest flaw being that if you didn't fit into the team, then you had a pretty miserable existence. It was a system in which all kinds of discrimination could thrive. I was lucky, though, and happy to be part of the team. Also, as I was still not very sure about being a doctor, I was more than happy to be on the bottom rung of a hierarchy. As a first year, pre-registration doctor, you did very little in the way of actually practising medicine. Your job was to make sure things ran smoothly: file notes, look for stuff, organise things etc. Many of my friends hated this and became quite despairing and disillusioned. I didn't mind and, generally, was quite cheerful about the whole thing.

I enjoyed the camaraderie. The hours were long and brutal; we spent most of our time in the hospital. Anything resembling a life was reduced to a small fringe around the edges. We tolerated this, as we had been sold the myth that once we were through this phase, things would become easier.

Although the hours were long, the workload wasn't as intense as it is nowadays. There was time to sit and drink coffee and arrange nights out, but, in many ways, the hospital was our whole world.

Nightshifts, in particular, were much less intense than they are now and there were also more doctors in the hospital overnight. If one person was particularly busy, we would all go and help them. We had the time and space to support each other emotionally, too.

In my second and third years, I chose general medicine: rotating through different specialties to gain experience in several before choosing one to pursue. It was during this period that things started to go wrong, and it was not a very happy time in my life.

Firstly, as a career choice, general medicine did not suit me. As I rotated through each specialty, all I realised was that I had no desire to do it and felt, at times, sick at the very idea of having to do it for the rest of my life. Furthermore, in order to specialise, you were required to sit a series of postgraduate exams. I was fed up with sitting exams. I only half-heartedly sat the first exam, and I kept on failing it.

I had also outgrown Dundee, since many of my friends had moved away. I felt left behind. More than that, I felt isolated, trapped, and restless.

Things came to a head on 2 January, 1997. I was working an old-fashioned on-call rota and had been on-call since the day before. This meant that I had started work at 8am on 1 January and worked until the ward round finished at 1pm on 2 January. I didn't get home until nearly three o'clock. I went to bed, but forced myself to get up after a couple of hours. If I stayed in bed, there was a danger that I might wake in the early hours of the morning and then not be able to get back to sleep again. This would mess with my sleep cycle for days.

I was miserable and felt nauseous from tiredness. What remained of the day was wet and dreary. My flatmate was away with her family for New Year. I sat in my living room feeling sorry for myself, and admitted that I hated what I was doing. My rotation finished in August and I would need to look for another job. I made a vow that I would knuckle down and study harder this time and pass the exam. In the interim, I would make enquiries about what jobs were out there. It wasn't a plan so much as a delaying tactic. I wasn't really confronting the main issue, which was that I was unhappy. I walked into the kitchen and, out of nowhere, found myself shouting.

'No,' I screamed, 'that's exactly what you won't do, for that is how people end up trapped in lives that they hate.'

Suddenly I was awake, energised, excited almost. I realised that I had a choice. But what could I do to get to a place where I would be happy? I wasn't even sure what I wanted or needed in order to be happy.

Eventually, an answer came to me. It seemed a bit crazy, but it had a strange kind of logic to it. If staying in and around Dundee, doing another job in general medicine and trying to pass my exam was exactly what I shouldn't do, then I should do the opposite. I should go somewhere else and do something different.

I had no idea what, but it seemed a good start. In front of me, my life seemed to shimmer. What had seemed so closed began to open up. The world was my oyster. Or the NHS hospitals of the UK were.

## January 2022: Almost a New Year's Resolution

The year started with the department under immense pressure. We were dealing with the Omicron wave of COVID, and we were already depleted after two years of the pandemic — which had come on top of the general exhaustion of trying to work in understaffed, overcrowded departments for years prior to its arrival. People were leaving and not being replaced. This made it harder for those that remained. It was a deep, wearying kind of exhaustion that reached right into your bones and couldn't be cured by a weekend off or even a holiday. Exhaustion was part of the new normal.

The combination of all these challenges had left us worn out and/or burnt out. There seemed no end to it. There were lots of NHS recovery plans but none of them discussed strategies to help the staff recover.

Nevertheless, I had started the year in an optimistic mood. Although COVID had knocked my life off-kilter, it was time to get some direction back. If I was doing that, I might as well think positively. This was unusual for me. I am cautious by nature. I'm not someone who hopes for the best or trusts that things will work out alright in the end.

Even so, I felt that it was important to focus on things that brought me happiness. At work, I was going to concentrate on projects concerning staff wellness. This was a subject that I was passionate about. Working on it brought me a lot of satisfaction, both professional and personal.

I would also rebuild aspects of my social life that had disappeared during the pandemic. I had become lazy regarding going out and meeting up with people. I would make more of an effort.

Also, I could go on holiday again, perhaps my favourite indulgence. The thought of wearing my summer clothes was another incentive to lose weight… to get healthier.

My diet-which-was-not-a-diet was going well. I was eating lots of lean protein and vegetables, making soup for lunch each day. More impressively, I had cut way back on carbohydrates. This was an almost unbelievable achievement. I am partial to cake, and I adore bread, pasta, potatoes and rice. To me, a meal isn't a meal without carbs. I had been eating wholemeal varieties since my teens when we were told that the best way to be healthy was to eat lots of fibre. The arrival of the Atkins diet demonised all carbohydrates, even the wholemeal ones, but I love them and the fact that I was willing to sacrifice them was a sign of my commitment.

About halfway through the month, I realised that I had not had an alcoholic drink since New Year. It occurred to me that I could do Dry January. I had had a couple of drinks on New Year's Day but I could just do an extra day in February. I was faintly amused at myself. Only recently, I had been astonished at people doing Dry January and now, here I was, fretting about the rules. I didn't drink much anyway. Even a couple of drinks left me feeling hungover and debilitated.

I increased my exercise. I was never what you might call sporty, but I did regular Zumba classes and walked home from work. I added in hand weights to some of the Zumba. I started walking to work, as well, and if I was going out to dinner, I would try to leave earlier and walk rather than use public transport.

I never weighed myself; I just went by how my clothes felt and looked. Disappointingly, they didn't feel or look any different by the end of the month. I was a bit despondent. But then again, everyone says it's much harder to lose weight when you're over fifty and menopausal. Surely you would expect to see some change by now, whispered a tiny voice in my head. You just have to be patient, I told myself. But I am an Emergency Medicine physician and patience doesn't come easily.

## Me and My Weight

At school, I had been one of the overweight children. I was lucky, and wasn't teased about it that much. But it was always there, something that became part of my identity. From time to time, we all had to get weighed in front of the class. Our weights were called out and recorded somewhere. It's the sort of thing that, like many things from the 70s, I imagine would not be done nowadays. I think we might even have guessed each other's weight beforehand, like some sort of awful fairground game, but I may just have imagined that part. Needless to say, I found the experience humiliating.

I dreaded PE. I just couldn't seem to do physical things as well as the others. I couldn't run very fast or do the high jump or even a forward roll. I didn't struggle academically. PE was the only place where I did not excel.

This was very stressful, but I was unable to articulate it. I feared that there was something defective about me. And that it was related to being fat. My fatness seemed to make me different from the other children. There was more of me, but it made me less than them.

My mum discussed my weight with the GP, who was an advocate of the 'eat less, move more, and try harder' school of thought. In a conversation that I have heard quoted many times, when my mum asked could there be something wrong with my glands perhaps, the reply was, 'Yes, her salivary glands.'

There were attempts to put me on diets and encourage more exercise but none of them seemed to work and they all fizzled out after a time. I continued to be the biggest girl in the class; perhaps, even, the biggest child.

I feel I had a normal relationship with food. But what constitutes a normal relationship with anything? Initially, it was intertwined with my relationship with my family, and as everyone's relationship with their family is complex, maybe, too, so was my relationship with food.

My earliest food memory dates from when I was about three years old. My mum and I would go once a week to my grandmother's house for Irish stew for lunch, though I think that back in the 70s, we were the kind of family who referred to the midday meal as dinner. The meal we ate in the evening was tea. That's another thing food is entwined with: class.

I was always excited to go to my granny's to eat, although, confusingly, I distinctly remember that I did not like Irish stew. I should add that this was not the only time I saw my grandmother. She lived in the same street; I saw her all the time. But there was something about the magic of going for food that turned that visit into a special occasion. And that is one belief about food that has stayed with me to this day. The addition of food to any gathering somehow elevates it. It turns the mundane into a celebration.

When I left home and lived in shared housing, most bad days could be made better by getting some nice food in. Sadness, badness and boredom were cured by sweets and cakes and crisps, dips and nice things from posh supermarkets. At some point in early adulthood, I realised that I was a social eater. So, despite my desire to lose weight, I couldn't lose my social life, nor forgo food, the glue that held it together and acted like fairy dust giving my days a little sparkle. Left on my own, I would eat much less. My enjoyment of food has always diminished if I'm not sharing it with someone.

Food may have been the cure to a bad day, but if I was really sad or worried or heartbroken, I would lose my appetite. All my failed relationships would result in a period of weight loss when they ended. Eating didn't just make me happy; I needed a certain level of happiness to want to eat.

Another reason food played a significant part in my upbringing was because my mother taught French cookery. As food was her livelihood, she viewed it as important. And from an early age, I also understood this importance. It sustained us in more ways than one; it was more than just nutrition. Food was a job, a currency, something to be studied, discussed, and perfected. Like many people, my mother showed her love through food. I am similar; I want to cook for people I care about.

My mother worked late at least one night a week. My father would collect me from school, and take me to Coleraine, about five miles away. I loved these trips, particularly in autumn. Those darkening days were magical. I still feel Christmas creeping in from about mid-October. I sense it in the mid-afternoon light as the low sun begins to set; I see it in the twisted silhouettes of leafless trees with their exposed birds' nests. On those October and November Wednesdays, my father and I looked for things to buy for Christmas, and my father loved Christmas. It was how he expressed his love.

Food also played a huge part in those Wednesdays. My father would cook me whatever I wanted for tea, often based on something that I had seen on television. He would make it for me and we would have it every Wednesday night until something else took my fancy. Things in favour included fish cakes and chips, spaghetti Bolognese and, bizarrely, French onion soup. I still love all of these to this day. So, Wednesdays, Christmas and food were the special bond I had with my father: our time, and the love that he had for me and the love that I had for him.

In retrospect, my diet was a bit more sophisticated than the average child growing up in Northern Ireland in the 70s, though I don't know if I particularly appreciated much of what I was given to eat. Due to my mum's work, she would occasionally bring leftovers home. Some of these I liked but some I didn't. Anything in aspic held particular horrors. From childhood I have always hated jelly, even the fruit stuff at children's parties.

My parents would often take me out to restaurants. Dining out was one of their indulgences. I was the type of child who would sit quietly with a colouring book and crayons. As I got older, would just sit quietly. I loved everything about going out for dinner. The food was important, but it was more than that: it was the atmosphere and the being looked after. My parents relaxed. That was the magic of restaurants: they made everyone happy and everything better. As soon as I started earning money of my own, going out for dinner was one of the things I spent it on.

Otherwise, we ate like everyone else: shepherd's pies and fish fingers, roast dinner on Sundays. From time to time, we would be short of money. My mother would come home and announce that we were on an economy drive. During one of these periods, when I was a teenager, one of the casualties was the Sunday roast. Instead, my mother went to the market and bought, for a ridiculously small amount of money, a huge bag of chicken wings which she put in the freezer. She marinaded them in ginger and honey and served them with brown rice. I loved that chicken and brown rice combination. I still think it might have been one of the best things I have ever eaten. For a few months, it became the highlight of my week. Then the economy drive ended, and the roast returned. I have tried to replicate the chicken and rice dish myself, but I have never been able to get it just right, just the way I remember.

It was more than just Sunday dinner. It was something exotic. This was another aspect of food that was becoming apparent to me in my late teens. Food was starting to represent new experiences, a whole world that existed outside my own, just waiting to be explored. Food, and indeed life, could be an adventure. I wanted to try it all.

So that was my relationship with food, or at least part of it. Food was love and connections and closeness. Food was magical, transformative. It could be both the comfort and safety of home and the adventure of far away. Was I too greedy? Did I eat too much? Maybe I did, maybe I didn't. All these years later, I don't think that I will ever know.

But I can see why dieting, denying all the joy that food brings, is so difficult, so hard to sustain. There is a certain kind of person who likes to say, from a place of judgement, that weight loss is simple: just eat less and move more. But it is so much more complicated than that: untangling all the threads that bind most of us to food, coupled with the potential to be utterly joyless. And I, for one, never wanted to lead a joyless life.

## February 2022: The New Normal

January seemed to go quickly. Maybe it was because I'd set myself goals and wasn't achieving them; it created the feeling that I was running out of time. I told myself to relax about my weight; I just needed to give it time.

The Omicron wave of COVID must have ended. It was hard to say when exactly these waves ended. There was no announcement. We just began to notice fewer cases and we talked about it less and less, until we hardly talked about it at all.

Or, more significantly, we began to talk about something else. Generally, as one problem diminished, a new one appeared to take its place. There was never a specific end to any issue. They all bled into each other. And when there was no specific emergency, we were back to having to deal with the permanent crisis of not having enough space. I can't remember when we had enough space; we had been treating patients in the corridors for years.

We had all chosen to work in an emergency department, but that didn't mean we wanted to work in a state of emergency all the time. The department was always busy. There were no quiet days anymore; only — and rarely — quieter ones. Anyway, one quiet day, or one day when the staffing was right, wasn't enough. We needed quiet stretches. Everything needs a fallow period in order to grow. We needed long, quiet periods to develop the department. We needed time to stop, to think and re-group.

But we couldn't; we were always firefighting. Or trying to hold back a vast tide, like lots of King Canutes. Sometimes, I was reminded of that story of the Dutch child who puts his finger in a leaking dyke to save the town from flooding. That's what it felt like we were doing: holding up an entire system from collapsing around us.

Occasionally, I would remember what the job was like when I fell in love with it. I wondered if anyone would fall in love with it now; some days, I struggled to see anything remaining of that old job. I could easily understand why so few people wanted to do Emergency Medicine training these days. Actually, it wasn't just Emergency Medicine training, it was all branches of medicine. Junior doctors were giving up and moving to Australia. I thought back to my own time in Australia and envied my younger self. It's hardly surprising that we have a retention crisis.

I organised some group reflective sessions. They were facilitated by one of our clinical health psychologists. They were to provide a time and a space for the team to share their experiences of working in the department.

We talked about how our day-to-day lives had been changed by COVID. No-one in the room was scared by COVID anymore, though we confessed that we had been. But it was as if it had done something to our lives, frayed them around the edges a little. People discussed little routines that they had lost, little things that they used to do that had brought them joy. Everyone admitted that they went out a lot less than they used to. It was as if, after we had all retreated to our houses during lockdown, we had never properly gone out again. It felt as if our lives had been taken apart and then roughly pushed back together in a sloppy, crude way. None of the joints and seams quite matched up and some pieces had been lost.

People seemed almost surprised when they remembered things that they no longer did. That's the thing about the details of our lives. It's so easy to lose sight of something if we just don't do it for a while. Once it would have felt strange but now the opposite is true. There was no grand ending, no farewell;, things just slipped from our lives. You never knew that one time would turn out to be the last time. And the loss seemed to have leached some colour or richness from our days.

It occurred to me that I never went out for coffee or had lunch on my own anymore. This used to be a ritual of mine. I liked to sit somewhere with my book and watch the world go by. Now the world was going by without me noticing it. It was an uncomfortable feeling.

Worst of all was that I had got used to not going out as much. I had grown comfortable with staying in. I told myself again that I needed to make more of an effort. I am, at heart, a people person.

I couldn't help thinking, ruefully, that not going out was more conducive to eating healthily. Maybe I would start trying to go out more when I managed to lose a bit of weight. I couldn't help but notice that my weight was now condemning me to my own, personal lockdown.

I was feeling good, though. I was sticking to my healthy eating plan. And I was walking everywhere, even though the weather was miserable.

I was enjoying not drinking. I felt quite sorry when January came to an end, so much so that I decided to continue. I went to a friend's birthday event and didn't drink. I sat on the tube on the way home feeling smug. I was grateful that I would not feel hungover the next day, and delighted by the calories that I had saved. That was one thing that pretty much every diet I had ever been on agreed about: alcohol was empty calories.

At the end of the month, I was going on holiday. It was in the UK, so I was not required to bring out all my holiday clothes which had been packed away since the pandemic began. I still wanted to look nice, though. I dug out a few things that I had not worn for ages. It was like meeting up with old friends. I was horrified when I tried them on. Most of them didn't fit. And the ones that did: just because they fitted didn't mean I should wear them. Now we were like old friends who find that they really don't have anything in common anymore.

Standing in my underwear, I was close to tears. To add insult to injury, I struggled to get out of the last thing I had put on; for a while I thought that I might have to cut myself out of it. Look at you, I thought, you're so fat that you need to perform minor surgery to get undressed.

How could this be? The menopause, I thought. Everyone warns you about the menopause and they're not wrong. What if I couldn't lose this weight? I thought back to the pandemic and what I had eaten. In the first wave, I was relatively good. I had stayed away from most of the free food that we had been given at work as I feared exactly this scenario. My resolve had slipped during the following waves. I didn't think that I had let myself go to this extent, but I must have done, because the old me was now just some distant mark on the horizon.

Why? I lamented. Why did I do this to myself? I would just have to diet harder. Except that I wasn't on a diet, I was just eating healthily. Maybe that was my problem. I needed to stop all this 'I'm just being healthy' nonsense and commit to being on a good old-fashioned diet, until I could get into my clothes again. I would be stricter when I came back. I would allow myself to enjoy my holiday first, though. Except that it was hard to enjoy as I didn't feel particularly good about myself.

One day in the hotel, I caught sight of myself in the mirror. Except for the day when I had tried on the clothes, I had been avoiding looking in mirrors. Even that day I had tried not to look for too long. But now I couldn't stop myself. The size of the mirror and the bright light in the room made my image even more pronounced than it had in my flat.

My weight and I had been locked in a perpetual struggle all my life. Sometimes I won, sometimes it did. But one thing remained constant, no matter who was winning, I always had an hourglass figure. Sometimes the hourglass was bigger than others, but that was the shape that I was. I looked at my reflection in morbid fascination: my waist had almost disappeared. This must be what the menopause belly looks like, I thought.

## 1997: A Leap of Faith

In the end, I realised that what I wanted, more than anything, was to go off, have fun and enjoy my life. This was considered quite a shocking decision. The term 'work/life balance' was not common in 1997. To many people, my thinking was incomprehensible; it amounted to career suicide.

But now I had a plan, I became proactive in pursuing it. As I have said, I had a terror of not having a job. It is interesting now, looking back, that despite my obvious unhappiness, it never once crossed my mind to take some time out. The thought of not working was just too frightening.

I had decided to get a job in Emergency Medicine, which was almost considered a rite of passage. Then, as now, there were lots of vacancies. Lots of people did a six-month stint; it was considered good experience. Also, much to my surprise, I realised that I enjoyed the acute aspect of general medicine. I liked seeing sick patients and managing them, much more than dealing with interminable ward rounds and outpatient clinics. In the early days, Emergency Medicine was the last thing that I thought that I would like. It had seemed too scary. I never imagined that I would relish it.

It was late January. Most places were not yet advertising their jobs for August or had just begun and had not filled any at this stage. This was no obstacle; I would just write to any hospital I liked the sound of and enquire as to vacancies. I happened to notice that Preston had only two left.

Gosh, Preston must be popular, I thought. This was not an incentive to apply as I felt success would be unlikely. But, perhaps, because it had stuck in my mind, I addressed an envelope to Royal Preston Infirmary before I realised what I had done. What the hell? I remember thinking, and then: I have lots of stamps and CVs, I might as well just send it. I sent off about twenty CVs — and the first place to get back to me was Preston, asking if I could come down for an interview the following Friday.

I caught the train from Dundee. It was one of those early February days when you can sense, in the wintry sun, a promise that spring is on the way. I read my book and looked out of the window as Scotland gave way to England. Mill towns began to appear amongst the fields and dry-stone walls. I had never been in this part of the world before.

I had an interview with the consultant in the department, Mr Mark James. I can't remember any of the questions he asked. I can, however, remember the light shining through the window behind him. It was late afternoon by then and the setting sun turned the sky and the room pink.

At the end of the interview, he said that he thought that I would be a good fit to the team, and he would like to offer me the job.

Immediately, I said yes. Mr James looked slightly surprised and asked me would I like to have more time to think about it, the weekend perhaps?

I said no. I told him, I was taking a leap of faith and I felt that, if you were going to take a leap of faith, it was best to do it quickly. Anyway, I added, I was a very decisive person. I often wonder if that was music to Mark James's ears. If there is one characteristic that is desirable in Emergency Medicine, it is decisiveness, and the more quickly you make a decision, the better.

I took a taxi to the station, gazing out of the window to get another glimpse at my future home and made the journey in reverse to Dundee. I finished my last few months there, happy and excited about the future. I was in no doubt that I had made the right decision. The time to leave came round quickly enough.

My parents were coming over to help me pack up my flat. A few days before they were due to arrive my father phoned, and we had a stupid argument about something. I can't even remember what. The next night, his best friend phoned me, around midnight, to tell me that my dad had dropped dead of a heart attack.

## March 2022: Performance

My early optimism began to wane. The department was frantically busy, without any specific disaster to blame it on. This was always a dangerous position to be in, as, again, attention would turn to our performance.

By performance, I mean that we were supposed to see and discharge ninety-five percent of patients within four hours. We could discharge them home or to somewhere else in the hospital. By March 2022, no hospital in the country was achieving anywhere near the ninety-five percent mark. The reasons for this were complex.

We had found ourselves in this position many times in the previous decade. It always boiled down to the same thing: we needed to work harder, faster or more efficiently, or all three. We needed to be more productive.

Sometimes the focus was on how long it took to see a patient after they arrived. If we could reduce that, surely that would speed up their progress through the department? Yes, it would. The problem was that we weren't slow to pick up new patients because we hadn't noticed them, nor were we wilfully ignoring them. We were slow to pick them up because we were already busy seeing all the other patients that had come in before them.

Surely, then, we could see those patients a bit faster and that would free us up to see the new patients more quickly? Yet again, there were multiple reasons why we couldn't do this. Emergency care needs time.

How quickly should we be processing a patient anyway? When I started Emergency Medicine, over twenty years ago, we were told that we should spend, on average, around one hour with a patient in the majors area. That was from the moment we picked them up until they either walked out the door or were handed over to another specialty. Obviously, some patients took longer, and some took less time, but the average was an hour.

Few people had mobile phones, alcopops were the threat to the youth that vaping is today, and the Spice Girls were all the rage. I make this last point to illustrate that we were living in a very different world back then. The demographics of patients visiting an emergency department have altered. Nowadays, many more patients have complex needs, and it follows that these patients will take longer to process. However, the one hour/patient notion has lingered. If staff are taking, on average, longer than that, they must be taking too long.

Also, we have many more patients coming into emergency departments than we did back then. This, incidentally, isn't just a British problem; it is replicated worldwide. Could we try and re-direct patients away from the emergency department? That would mean fewer patients coming in, and fewer to attend to.

Now we're deep into King Canute territory here. Firstly, it's a myth that most people who come to an emergency department don't need to be there. Some don't, but lots do. Even people that technically don't, don't have anywhere else to go as the services they need are no longer available.

Also, in numerous discussions around attendance figures, patients who didn't need to be there were sometimes conflated with patients who were seen and discharged. The assumption was that if you needed to be there, it followed that you should be admitted. Many patients who were discharged *had* needed to be there. They had often received a lot of care in between arriving and going home. In fact, this was what enabled us to discharge them. Moreover, this aspect of the work was what we considered our jobs to be, and was an area in which we took a great deal of satisfaction and pride. It was one of the things that made us want to come to work in the morning. Unfortunately, it was one of the time-consuming parts of the job.

And here is another problem: it often takes much longer to discharge a patient than it does to admit them. But time was the one thing we didn't have. We were supposed to be seeing the patients faster, but sending them home always took longer.

Anyway, we couldn't send all of them home; some needed to come into hospital. And this caused another problem. We had no beds. So, of course, patients ended up waiting in the department for hours. Our trolley spaces would quickly be taken up and we would have to start seeing patients in the corridor and anywhere else that we could find. On bad days, we even had to see patients in ambulances.

Again, this was a nationwide issue. Many hospitals were in a much worse position than we were. But it was an awful thing to have to do. Truly awful. I think it's hard for anyone who doesn't have to work in those conditions, day in and day out, to understand how completely distressing it is.

Every day you feel that you are doing something wrong, something that goes against everything you believe. Intellectually, although you know that it isn't your fault, but the fault of the system, it isn't the system that has to look patients in the eye as they lie on trolleys for hours. It isn't the system that has to deliver what you know, in your heart of hearts, to be poor care.

The effect that this had on the staff was rarely discussed and definitely not discussed in detail. It was less important than trying to find solutions to how we could see patients more quickly, despite the fact that one thing that could undoubtedly help us to see patients more quickly — and efficiently — was to ensure that we had the space to do it in.

We persisted in trying to find a way of making something work. Perhaps this is just human nature. Sometimes it's hard to see a solution when you don't give yourself any space or time to stand back and look at problems objectively. But space and time were luxuries we didn't have. Even pointing this out was risky. Being so negative all the time was risky. Emergency Medicine is full of problem-solvers. We are constantly trying to find solutions and demonstrate a 'can do' attitude.

Things were also complicated by the fact that on some days we would, by chance, have enough beds in the hospital but still we wouldn't meet the target. So, our poor performance wasn't only to do with beds. Could we work out what had happened on those days and use that to direct us?

Often, we didn't have enough doctors. Like every hospital in the country, we had huge rota gaps. We invested inordinate amounts of time trying to recruit but, as this was a national crisis — in fact, an international one — this had a very poor yield. Anyway, recruitment wasn't the main problem, it was retention. No-one wanted to do the job and who could blame them?

We could do nothing to improve the job. Many factors, such as pay, were completely out of our control. We were spinning round this never-ending, ever-decreasing circle. And we were all so tired. Many of us had been tired trying to deal with this Kafkaesque carnival since before the pandemic. COVID had made things worse, but it seemed that everyone had forgotten about that and we were expected to behave as if it had never happened, to perform as if we had never gone through it. Perhaps that was one of the reasons that we failed to achieve the target, even when we had enough beds. We were just too exhausted. But that never featured in the analysis of the figures. And even if it had, I'm not sure that we could have solved it with an action plan.

I was tired, too. Of course, I'd been fed up with the pressure around performance for some time. But now I was starting to feel physically tired too, exhausted in a way I had never felt before. Not every day but more often than not. I was really beginning to hate the menopause. I was finding it harder to cope with everything, harder to deal with it mentally and physically. I wasn't burnt out — or at least I didn't think that I was — but I was maybe just a little singed around the edges.

And then there was my weight. Despite my best efforts, I still didn't seem to be able to lose any. Occasionally, I thought that, if anything, I might look bigger. Could the menopause be that diabolical? No, I would just have to be stricter. But how, how can you be stricter? whispered a little voice; you're being so strict already. There's always room for improvement, I told it firmly. Just like in the department, I needed to try harder.

## 1986: Summer

In 1981, I went to a girls' grammar school and became the fat one there. Amazingly, once again, I did not experience any bullying about my weight. I was in a year group in which there was very little bitching.

In the earlier years, at least, weight was not talked about very much. Certainly, there was no extreme dieting, no-one with eating disorders. We just seemed to accept the complete package of ourselves. There was not much obsessing over isolated body parts. You were either fat or thin or somewhere in between. This was before plastic surgery became so accessible. We didn't talk about boob jobs or lip fillers. From memory, most of us just had normal arms. I recently watched an old episode of *Top of the Pops* and was shocked that the female singers also just had normal arms.

Of course, it was still best to be thin. But I was fat. And even though no-one ever said anything, I always sensed that awareness hanging there, unspoken. I hated it. I also hated that I couldn't dress like my friends.

One particularly cruel irony was that I loved clothes and I loved fashion. I still do. Retail therapy specifically is one of my guilty pleasures. Back in the early 80s, I wanted to wear the same clothes as my friends. And, as this was the 80s, this included items such as ra-ra skirts and pedal pushers. Some might wryly say that I had a lucky escape, but my thirteen-year-old self-longed for a ra-ra skirt with a desire which hurt. And I wanted to be able to wear shorts in the summer like everyone else.

Then, finally, along came 'that summer'. As an adult, I have sometimes become friendly with other women who would reveal that they too had been the fat child in their school. And many of them had had their own version of 'that summer'.

For me, it was 1986. I was sixteen, and had just sat my O-levels. My mother had ordered clothes from one of the catalogues that mothers always ordered clothes from in the 70s and 80s. Most of them were horrible even before I tried them on. They were the sort of clothes I wore because I had to, not because I wanted to. There were a few things that I had chosen with hope. But they didn't fit or, if they did, they looked awful. It felt like the clothes were rejecting me and not the other way around.

My mother had received, as a free gift, a set of bathroom scales. Or perhaps I have imagined the scales as a gift; maybe we always had them and I had just ignored them. I found weighing myself distressing. Anyway, that night, somehow, I was persuaded to get on the scales. And it was traumatic, very traumatic. I went to bed crying, all thoughts of my O-level results forgotten. I had something much bigger to worry about: myself.

So, I put myself on a diet, as opposed to being put on one: self-motivated and, also, self-designed. Looking back, it is almost laughable, as it consisted of various items that today are most definitely thought of as kryptonite for dieters: foods so heinously terrible that they are avoided like the plague. Basically, my diet contained an awful lot of carbohydrates. But this was the 80s. Carbohydrates were not the enemy; fat was.

My mother had recently had to have her gallbladder removed. Waiting for her operation, she had been unable to eat anything containing fat as it left her in agony. She had been forced to develop her own low-fat diet to avoid pain, and the side effect had been weight loss.

Along with the prevailing wisdom that fat was the enemy, there was also a feeling that meat was not that good for you and vegetarianism was a healthier option.

I had Weetabix with semi-skimmed milk, followed by a slice of dry toast for breakfast. Lunch was two medium-sized baked potatoes (actually, just microwaved) with no butter and low-fat cottage cheese. For my evening meal, I had exactly the same. I had an apple for a snack in the morning and again in the afternoon. Finally, before bed, I had two digestive biscuits. On Sundays, for a bit of variation, I allowed myself some roast chicken, no skin. I ate the same thing every day all summer. I never cheated, never wavered and I refused every sweet I was offered.

This diet revealed a lifelong character trait: a cast-iron will. And my life was not without its temptations. At the time, my parents owned a guest house and so spent their days churning out all manner of delicious things: fry-ups for breakfast, cottage pie for lunch and fish and chips for tea. But I sat there, with the smell of frying bacon and chips, rigidly sticking to my dry toast and cottage cheese. If I set my mind to something, I would do it.

What is most remarkable, particularly in these carb-hating days, is that it worked. Nowadays, more than twenty years since I first heard about the Atkins diet, I would never consider eating four baked potatoes in an ordinary day, never mind as an attempt to lose weight. Even though I know that it once worked. It worked a treat, in fact.

Initially, I was disappointed. At my first weigh-in, I had lost a mere 2lbs. I looked at the scales in despair. Of course, all good dieters will say that slow and steady is how you do it. But I didn't want slow and steady. I wanted fast and immediate. I nearly gave in there and then, but my cast-iron will had been activated. The next week I lost another 2lbs, and another two a week later. That was nearly half a stone and that, somehow, felt substantial. I was also beginning to feel a little different in myself.

I had a job in a local department store. At first, I felt self-conscious going into the break room and eating only an apple. I needn't have worried. The store had a number of female employees, and most of them were no strangers to dieting. They had seen it all before. But as the summer progressed, and I persisted, they began to take notice.

'Gosh, Heidi, you're losing the weight,' someone said one day.

'I was thinking that,' said another. 'I saw you from behind when I came in this morning and didn't recognise you for a moment.'

It was intoxicating, all these positive comments about my weight. I wanted to lose more. My O-level results came and went. I did well. But my academic success did not bring me nearly as much pleasure as my diminishing size.

On and on the summer went. And on and on, losing weight, I went. By the end, I had lost over a stone. And it made a huge difference to my sixteen-year-old appearance. I was transformed. It was rare for me to go into work and not get some sort of compliment about my size. It was glorious.

To keep the 'all you have to do is eat less and move more, it's that simple' brigade happy, it is worth saying that I was also moving more. At the start of my diet, I had also realised that if I wanted to lose weight, I would have to start exercising. So I started running. Trying to run would be a fairer way of describing it. Of course, as it was the 80s, it was referred to as jogging.

I decided that I would go jogging every evening. Obviously, when I started, I was not that good. 'I couldn't run the length of myself,' as the phrase goes. In all honesty, I think I managed about three lengths of myself before becoming red-faced, sweaty and so out of breath that I had to stop.

But I had made my mind up and so, every evening I ran, and every evening I ran a little bit further than the night before. What's more, I began to enjoy it.

## April 2022: Not a Cause for Celebration

The first time it happened was in April. It was one of those early spring days that has a freshness about it. I yearned to be happy and carefree, to feel like me again. I couldn't remember the last time I had felt like me. I wasn't even sure what that meant anymore.

It would be simplistic to say that the real me was happy and carefree. It was in my nature also to be wry and cynical, but I had the sense that something was amiss inside me. Something had happened to the proportions. I just assumed it was to do with getting older.

There was an anxiety somewhere, a faint hum in the distance. I couldn't pinpoint where it was coming from. Had COVID done this? Had I always carried around a little fear that something dreadful might happen? A fleeting little fear, that I was able to push to the farthest part of my mind and expel from my consciousness? Perhaps COVID had made that fear a reality.

Let's face it, dreadful things do happen. Most of the time they don't, but that doesn't mean that they can't. I should know this better than anyone. At work, I see dreadful things every day. Actually, that is an exaggeration. Some days, I'm not even working a clinical shift; I'm just in my office. But there are times when doctors face truly catastrophic situations. Times when you have to tell someone that their relative has just died or is just about to. Times when you have to deliver some type of terrible diagnosis: that a patient's symptoms indicate something life-threatening, or life-changing. That sort of dreadful. I have seen it often enough for it to send a shiver — no, something sharper than a shiver: a slice — through my soul.

Maybe that's why so many of us in the emergency department develop such a dark sense of humour — to create a place where we can hide those memories. Our own secret place where we can bury the bodies.

Years ago, when I worked in Australia, I spent some time working in the ITU. One weekend, we started with seven patients, all of whom were predicted to die. 'Maybe we should take a bet,' I said, 'as to who will last the longest.' It was a throwaway line that I would hesitate to say to anyone other than a doctor. In isolation it sounds horrible: flippant, mocking. But it wasn't like that. It was a way of trying to deal with the situation, of coping with all that horror. If you can laugh it down, it won't defeat you.

I would have immediately forgotten that I said it, but I was working with a very junior doctor, who seized upon it and held onto it all weekend. I could see how the line was working inside her, how it was weaving its way into her psyche. Sometimes you just need something tough to cling to.

By Monday morning, all the patients were dead. A few days later, the junior doctor came to find me. Relatives of one of the patients who had died had come back with chocolate to thank everyone for their care. She had brought some down for me. She was insistent that I got some of it. It's another example of how food can say something for which we don't always have the vocabulary. We gave each other a little hug. Sometimes you just need something tender to cling to.

On that April morning, I felt like I was still waiting for something so that I could feel happy again. But I wanted to feel happy now. So, I decided that I was going to wear some of my old clothes: things I hadn't worn for a while; clothes that I had been instinctively avoiding. I had been waiting until I had lost weight. But, I reasoned, I must have lost a bit of weight by now.

I started off gently: a pair of leggings and a long black top that reached almost to my knees. The problem was that the top was made from a jersey-style material that seemed much stiffer than normal jersey. Getting into it was a struggle, but I persevered. Getting dressed in the morning shouldn't be a fight, whispered a little voice in my head. Yes, well, that might be true but, the reality was that every day was a fight. Working felt like a battle; the Emergency Department permanently resembled a war zone.

I won the getting-dressed skirmish and checked in the mirror. My overall appearance was lumpy. The top definitely looked tighter than it had previously. But at least I'd got it on. I did not feel that this was much of a cause for celebration. I stretched the material to loosen it, pulled it down over my knees and then lifted each knee up and outwards to create more space. That looks better, I told myself. I felt a bit more like me again.

At work, I went to buy a coffee and saw someone I knew. Pre-COVID, when you went to the coffee shop, you always bumped into someone you knew. Now you could go for days and not run into anyone. But, this morning, I met a colleague whom I had not seen for ages.

'You look well,' she said.

I smiled and thanked her. But, strangely, she kept on repeating it and I didn't understand why. I didn't look that well. There was something else, a pause after she spoke, and there was something unsaid in the pause. I had the notion that I was supposed to fill it. Was I missing something?

At the counter, I ran into another acquaintance.

'Hello,' she said, brightly. 'I didn't know that you were expecting. Congratulations.'

I felt myself go red. Oh, my God, she thinks I'm pregnant. I am so fat that she thinks I'm pregnant. How humiliating, how totally humiliating.

'I'm not pregnant,' I muttered. 'It's the opposite. I'm menopausal.'

Neither of us knew what to say.

'Bloody menopause,' I added, trying to break the tension.

After I got my coffee, I scurried back to my office. I did not want to meet a third person who thought that I was pregnant. I had had enough embarrassment for the day. The office was empty, and I scrutinised myself in the little mirror. It was not full length, but I got a view of about half my body. I saw myself face on and then turned to the side. I supposed the way my fat was distributed did make me look like I had a bump.

I sat down and did not leave the office until it was time to go home.

I really didn't want to see anyone else. More to the point, I didn't want anyone else to see me.

How could I have grown so fat that I now looked pregnant? Behind the humiliation, something else bubbled: despair, maybe. I had been dieting pretty hard for three months now and for what?

I walked home as quickly as I could. I tried to catch a glimpse of myself in each shop window. I definitely had something that looked like a bump. I wanted to stop and scrutinise myself but couldn't, for obvious reasons.

When I got home, it was time for my Zumba class. During lockdown, one of my instructors had taken her classes online and continued to run some of them that way. I now did a mixture: some classes in the gym and a few from my flat. I had bought some hand weights of varying sizes and generally did the class holding some light ones. I selected a heavier set. Desperate times call for desperate measures. I looked at myself on the screen. How had I not noticed that I looked pregnant?

I suppose it was because I didn't spend that much time looking at myself and when I did, I was face on. But now that I knew I had a huge bump, it was hard not to see it. I twisted and turned during the class, trying to catch a side view of myself.

As soon as the class finished, I went to the mirror. I felt foolish: this is what happens when you take your eye off the ball. The ball in this case being me or — should I say? — my belly. I turned this way and that, studying myself from every angle. I couldn't believe that I was the shape that I was: it was all wrong; I was all wrong. All my life I had battled with my weight but, even at my largest, I had never looked like this.

My entire shape had changed. All my life, no matter my size, my waist was always smaller than the rest of me. I had had an hourglass figure but now I was an apple, to use the language of countless women's magazines and of Trinny and Susannah, from *What Not To Wear*, who used to tell us how to dress.

I needed Trinny and Susannah now, as I had no idea how to dress this. And by 'this', I meant me. Curse you, menopause, curse you, I thought. I started to cry. I wasn't just crying because my belly was so big that I looked pregnant; there was grief in there, too. I had had a love/hate relationship with my shape down the years, but it was my shape, it was me — and, now it had gone, I felt like I had lost a bit of myself. I feared that I would never get it back again. It was gone forever. This was the new normal. And, as with the new normal at work, it was like the old normal, just a lot worse.

I had no idea how to be this shape. Not that you can't look good as an apple. I distinctly remembered that Trinny and Susannah had had lots of tips; I just hadn't paid that much attention as they hadn't applied to me. Also, I had a vague idea it was all about making the most of your legs and, even at my smallest, I had chunky legs, to put it kindly.

But more than how I looked, my body shape didn't *feel* like me. You're going to have to get used to it, I told myself, severely. Anyway, apple shape or no apple shape, you're going to have to be a smaller apple because you can't go on looking pregnant.

Perhaps I've invented a new body type, the melon, I thought.

I was just going to have to diet harder. 'But how?' whispered the tiny voice in my head. 'You're already dieting so hard, what else can you do?'

I was going to have to reduce my portion size again. Also, I was still eating a slice of wholemeal toast in the morning and some wholemeal brown rice with my evening meal. I'm going to have to give up the carbs, I told myself.

No! Not the carbs!

But you're so fat, you look pregnant, I admonished myself. I remembered the stinging humiliation from earlier.

Ditch the carbs.

## 1997: Belonging

When my father's friend told me that he had died, I screamed. I can't remember what, exactly; it might have been, 'No, no, you're lying.'

When people hear horrendous, life-changing news, they broadly break down into two groups: those who sit silently as they process the information and those who scream or shout. My next thought was, 'Gosh, who'd have known you'd turn out to be a screamer?' Then I had an image of a great ship trying to turn, tilting, and nearly falling over, righting itself and continuing. For years, I would wonder about that image. It seemed to have come from somewhere deep in my subconscious.

My father had died from a massive heart attack and subsequent cardiac arrest. It was totally unexpected. He was fifty-eight, well, and had had no symptoms. Or perhaps he had and had just never admitted them to anyone, even himself. As I was to see, time and again, people will deny all sorts of symptoms, even the most obvious: symptoms that you would think it would be impossible to ignore. But it's remarkably easy to ignore something that you don't want to be there.

I went home for my father's funeral and then on to my new job in Preston, starting just a week late. There were suggestions that, perhaps, it was too soon, but I was keen to go. I felt that I needed some normality in order to start processing my grief.

But what normality? I had lost a close family member, moved to a town where I did not know anyone, and started a different job. These are listed as three of life's major stressors and I was experiencing them all at once.

For the first time ever, I was very kind to myself. Each night, I told myself that I was a marvel, a wonder. The fact that I had got through the day was a miracle. And, in its own odd way, something more than a miracle: it was enough. I told myself each day that whatever I had done was enough.

I remember that year in Preston very fondly. I was looked after, cared for and, in many ways, loved by the department. They all held me safe.

I was now one of those people who had lost a parent, which at twenty-six years of age, was unusual amongst my peers. I had become a member of a special club, a club I neither wanted nor expected to be in.

Looking back, I can see that it was not just my colleagues that supported me. It seemed as if Emergency Medicine rose up and embraced me, too. The chaos of the department matched the chaos inside me. When I was at work, the job somehow balanced me out and soothed me. In those early days of grief, the Emergency Department was the only place where I felt that I belonged.

I had only been working in Preston for a few weeks when I had a week off and I went back home to Ireland. Everything seemed odd and disjointed. On the Sunday afternoon, I went for a walk along the beach. I had walked the beach ever since I was a teenager. It was a place that always brought me a lot of joy, and also comfort when I was upset about anything.

As I walked, I began to realise that I no longer felt I belonged anywhere. I had spent the last nine years of my life in Dundee, but I had emotionally disconnected from there long before I physically left. I had only been in Preston for just over a month and so did not feel any sense of belonging there. And now I realised that I no longer felt as if I belonged at home. I referred to it as home as I had no other word to describe it. I wondered when this dislocation had happened. Was it after my father had died or had it happened earlier, and I was only just beginning to notice now?

I looked out at the sea and thought that it, too, didn't belong anywhere. I remembered something that I had been told as a child during a school assembly. The sea we saw on our beach was the same sea that stretched all across the world. The waves breaking on the shore could well contain water that had lapped against the shores of all sorts of far and distant lands.

The sea belongs both nowhere and everywhere, I thought. Maybe I, too, could belong nowhere and everywhere. The idea brought with it a notion of freedom. Using the same logic that had got me out of Dundee, I realised that what I should do was travel as far as the sea could take me.

I wondered where that was: what was the farthest point from Portrush? Somewhere in the Pacific Ocean, perhaps even New Zealand? In the end, I decided that I would go to Australia. It maybe wasn't the farthest place, but it was still pretty far. Also, I knew someone who lived in Melbourne. Yes, I thought, that's what I'll do, I will go to Melbourne. And, having a plan, I immediately began to feel better.

I went back to Preston and began to settle down. Then along came the end of October. One afternoon, I was off work and lying on my bed, reading, when I suddenly felt a shiver of excitement and thought: Christmas is coming. Then I remembered that my father was dead. In my mind, Christmas and my father were inseparable. And my next thought was: how the hell am I supposed to get through Christmas without him? Followed by: why am I only realising this is a problem now?

It is very hard to hide from Christmas. It's just everywhere you go. It's unavoidable: the lights, the music, the adverts on TV. In December, people start saying, 'It doesn't feel like Christmas.' What? Are you mad? It doesn't feel like anything else! Also, the fact that people say it every year means that it is almost a Christmas tradition in itself.

It took me three attempts to do my Christmas shopping. On the first occasion, I took the bus into Preston town centre, stood for a few moments, decided I couldn't go through with it, turned around and got straight back on the bus. The second time I got as far as a shop, where they were playing Judy Garland singing *Have Yourself a Merry Little Christmas*. I burst into tears and gave up for that day. Finally, the Friday before Christmas, I told myself I had no choice and forced myself.

After I had done my shopping, I sat on a bench by the market and bought a cup of coffee from a van. I thought that I would be safer outside and not trapped inside a café with all the decorations. I was wrong. It was very Christmassy, with lights and tinsel and a great big tree. There may even have been a Salvation Army band, but I could have just made that bit up, layered it on top of the truth over time, as I turned a memory into a story.

I looked at this Christmas extravaganza, but I was too drained to move away. An elderly woman came and sat beside me and made some comment about needing to rest her legs. Then, she must have asked me how I was, and I found myself telling her. It was one of those times when you end up telling a stranger absolutely everything. I told her how my father had recently died, how he had loved Christmas, how I was dreading it and had only just done my Christmas shopping.

Then she told me her story. Her first husband had died many years before, leaving her with a seven-year-old daughter and very little money. She had really struggled the first Christmas, but she had managed. She had gone on to meet someone else, married again, and been very happy. That first Christmas had been hard, though. 'But I got through it, love, and so will you,' she said. I burst into tears and then she gave me a big hug and sat there holding me until I stopped crying. I always think back on it as one of the most Christmassy things ever to happen to me.

I learned something that year, and that is not everyone loves or even likes Christmas. I had joined another new club: the people-who-struggle-with-Christmas club. I was to be a member of this one for quite a number of years to come.

## April 2022: Getting Older

My tiredness was worse. Or maybe I was just more aware of it. I was also irritable: constantly tetchy. Maybe I was perpetually hangry. I was sticking to my new, super-improved diet. Whether or not it was having any effect remained to be seen.

I started watching myself in shop windows, but the fleeting glimpses showed no change. I scrutinised myself in the mirror: no change. In rare moments of optimism, I told myself that perhaps my belly only looked so big because I was losing weight everywhere else. The menopausal belly fat was just particularly resistant. I would simply have to persevere.

I also needed to be more careful about what I was wearing. I had, perhaps, been too optimistic about what I had worn on 'pregnancy day', as I now thought of it. Now that I had become so aware of my large belly, I began to think that everything made me look pregnant. In the end, I stuck to a few of the old favourites: large, stretchy, comfortable and mostly black.

At the end of the month, it was my birthday. I went home to Ireland for the week. On the day, we all went out for dinner. Afterwards, Sarah and her boyfriend went to the pub, and I went home with my mother. I felt sad, not because I was not going to the pub; I could have gone if I had wanted to. I felt sad because I didn't want to. Once upon a time, all I wanted was to go out and now all I wanted was to get home. I felt far too tired to go to the pub. And far too fat. I suppose I just have to accept that I'm getting old, I told myself as I got ready for bed.

# Faustian Pact

Eventually, the summer of 1986 ended, and it was time for me to go back to school. I couldn't help feeling excited. I had a whole new audience to show my weight loss to. Oh, how I relished those first few days, walking up to people, seeing the look of astonishment on their faces. Girls I hardly knew came up to compliment me, tell me how well I looked.

I could join in the conversations about clothes. I was able to partake fully in quite possibly the most exciting thing ever to happen to Coleraine: the arrival of Top Shop. I was able to try clothes on, just like everyone else. We tried clothes on for the fun of it; none of us could afford anything.

I couldn't remember ever being so happy. Little did I realise that I had signed my equivalent of a Faustian pact. As all the books, experts or anyone who has ever dieted will tell you, losing weight isn't the hardest part: that's keeping it off.

And what an epic battle it is. It's like something from Norse mythology. Dieting has its own particular tactical manoeuvres, and I have always been at some point of engagement with them: either on a diet or gaining weight or deciding to diet or about to start a diet. Even not dieting is a dieting stratagem. It doesn't mean that dieting has gone away; it just means it's in abeyance, but will, at some point, be followed by 'deciding to go on a diet'.

Possibly the most dangerous is the 'about to start a diet' part. Then you have your personal equivalent of Shrove Tuesday. You finish all the 'naughty' food in the house, including your emergency chocolate stash.

Then the fateful day arrives and you have a breakfast of black coffee, or herbal tea, and dry toast or porridge made with semi-skimmed milk or bacon and eggs (no bread) or egg white omelette or berries with Greek yoghurt and toasted seeds or absolutely nothing at all because you have chosen intermittent fasting or whatever else the latest diet advice says you should be eating in order to lose weight.

Over the years, in my battle with my weight, sometimes it has won and other times I have. Perhaps I've never had a resounding victory, but I've at least forced a draw. The problem is that it's not just my weight that's gone up and down, but my self-esteem, along with my pleasure in life and my pleasure in being me. I'm constantly chasing those compliments that I received, chasing the approval and the euphoria I felt.

When I'm smaller, all is right with the world and when I'm bigger, I'm unsettled, discontent. I feel disapproval and rejection. I wear my life like tightly fitting clothes, uncomfortable and restricting. I've been big and I've been smaller, but never quite as small as I thought that I should be.

What was worse was the goal posts kept changing. When I was at school, a size 12 was considered normal and a size 10 skinny. But then size 8 became the new size 10. So, in order to be thin, I had to go even further than before and then sustain it. Of course, size 8 didn't stay as the marker for skinny forever. In time, there was heroin-chic and the rise of size zero.

All the images in magazines, pop videos, TV and film showed very thin women. These very thin women were the ones deemed beautiful, who were succeeding at life, worthy of love and eventually just normal. In TV land, the teachers, waitresses, girls in nightclubs etc were all a certain size: a size that was getting further and further away from the size I was or even the size I could achieve with a certain amount of effort.

Fatness was to be pitied or ridiculed or despised. Think of Monica in *Friends*; think of Bridget Jones. Perhaps Bridget Jones was trying to put a positive spin on things. Despite her fears of being fat and, therefore, unworthy of love, she managed in the end. But that message didn't, for example, reach

Renée Zellweger who had to fatten up to play the role and began to slim down again as fast as she could when it was over. She couldn't bear to stay that size for a moment longer than she had to.

Even when my friends all told me that I didn't need to lose weight, that I looked fine as I was, they all thought that *they* needed to lose weight. They were all on diets, even the ones who were smaller than me.

I can remember what size I was at most times of my life, and where I was in the lifecycle of a diet. My size has burrowed itself into all my memories, both good and bad. If I was unhappy, I generally viewed my size as a cause. It never once occurred to me to think of it as an effect of what might be happening in my life.

I was a junior doctor in the late 90s. Now, there are aspects of that job that I loved and many reasons why I would rather have been a junior doctor back then, than nowadays. But the truth is, we worked insane hours.

My first job had the traditional on-call system, in which we started at 8am or 9am, worked all day and then were resident on-call in the hospital from 5pm to 8am the next morning. Sometimes we were lucky and got some sleep and other times we weren't and were awake all night. Then we worked the next day from 8am to 5pm. I did this once or twice a week, depending on how many people were on leave. It was brutal and unremitting.

We were also working in conditions where we had to deal with some challenging circumstances. At that time, it was not fashionable to talk about the emotional impact of the job. To some, it was dangerous; it was considered harmful to 'dwell' on things. The prevailing attitude was that we just needed to get on with it. Anything less than that was a failing. There was a fair amount of bravado; no-one wanted to admit that they might be struggling. We all affected a hard exterior to get by.

In the time I had off work, I did what many of my peers did — I went to the pub or out for dinner. As one of our team said, 'Who needs a car when you are a junior doctor? You're either working or drunk.' This was not particularly conducive to a healthy lifestyle and, no doubt, took its toll.

For me, there was no way I was able to do it and not put on weight. My diet was shocking, and I found it hard to make time for exercise. And so, the inevitable happened and my weight began to creep up. And with that came the equally inevitable disappointment in myself, and, at times, self-hatred.

But what was I to do? I wanted to make the most of the scraps of time that I had for me, in amongst the hours of work in an increasingly frayed life. I wanted to have fun and socialise, and this was the only way that I could think of doing it.

As a child, I had always believed that my weight made me not good enough. Now, as an adult, every failure to lose weight reinforced that belief. I blamed myself entirely for the predicament I found myself in. Round and round I went, trying to lose weight and failing. And as the blame grew, so did the shame.

## May 2022: Dropping Like Flies

My time off had done nothing to help either my tiredness or my mood. The department was still busy, and the pressure showed no sign of letting up. I had to drag myself in every day. I was so weary of it all.

Then things got worse. My department has ten consultants in Adult Emergency Medicine and one in Paediatric Emergency Medicine. Within a short period of time, five consultants took sick.

'We're dropping like flies,' we began to say, only half-jokingly.

None of the injuries and ailments seemed connected; they were just a random selection of things that, unfortunately, were all occurring simultaneously. But, beneath the surface, I felt they told a different story. We were all falling apart. I could hardly ever remember my colleagues being sick and now five were unwell at once. I became fixated on this.

One of my colleagues suffered a stress fracture. 'What bigger metaphor do we need?' I kept repeating to anyone who would listen. 'We are all breaking with the stress. There is only so much that our bodies can take.'

With so many people off, everything became harder. I was tired all the time, as were my colleagues. We needed a new word to describe how we felt. But there wasn't one. I could only express how tired I felt by putting the word 'so' in front of the word 'exhausted.' Some days, I needed more than one, as I was so, so exhausted.

We tried to get cover, but no-one was interested, and the only option was to battle on. It wasn't just a physical tiredness, but a mental one too. I felt that I could no longer cope with the department. I began to feel anxious in work. This had never happened to me before. Work had always been my safe space, my comfort zone. Now it felt as if it was turning on me. Sometimes I felt fearful of it. I began to dread going to work. I had the sense that my life was spinning out of control.

A friend said that they thought I was burnt-out. Maybe I was; it had crossed my mind. I had spent the last few years dedicating myself to staff wellness. I knew all about burnout. But there's a world of difference between knowing something and feeling it. I would be a classic example of someone too busy considering the wellness of others to look after her own.

Maybe I was in some sort of pre-burnt-out state. This was ridiculous and just splitting hairs. Burnt-out or pre-burnt-out, I should do something about it. But what? I couldn't reduce my hours. Half my colleagues were off sick and we couldn't get cover for them. I couldn't add to the problem.

Even as I thought this, I heard warning bells. These were exactly the thought patterns of burnt-out people: that martyred prioritising of other things over their own health. The idea that I would walk away from it all, especially now, seemed outrageous. I just couldn't bring myself to do it.

And if I did, what would I walk away to? The idea of doing nothing also terrified me. Again, a little warning bell rang. The other side of the coin to 'the department can't do without me' is 'I can't do without the department'.

Anyway, it wasn't just work that was getting me down. Something else was on my mind. And that something was my weight.

I decided to do something that I had never done in all my long years of dieting. I decided to buy some diet supplements. An advert kept popping up on my internet feed and they sounded too good to be true.

Yes, said that little warning voice. That's because they probably are.

A few days later, at a Zumba class in the gym, I thought I could make out my old shape again in the mirror. If I only kept up my efforts, with the help of the diet supplements, I could be myself again.

# 1998: As Far as the Sea Can Take Me

I was very happy during my year in Preston, and I might well have ended up staying in the north-west, if it hadn't been for a slightly drunken conversation one evening in the pub opposite the hospital.

'I'm going to go and work in Australia,' I announced to everyone.

'Bet you won't,' they said. 'You'll end up working here forever.'

'Or you might get to Bolton or maybe Manchester,' someone added.

Bet I will get to Australia, I thought; I'll show you.

That spirit was still upon me when I got back, slightly tipsy, to my room in the doctors' residence. And so, I phoned the switchboard and asked to be put through to the international directory. I knew one person in Melbourne and had once heard her mention the name of a hospital there, St Vincent's. That was all I knew about it, its name.

I asked for St Vincent's number and called the main switchboard. It was late at night in England and so it would be morning there. I asked to be put through to the Emergency Department and then asked to be put through to the doctor in charge. I was put through to Mr Andrew Dent, who was indeed the doctor in charge. Anyone who has ever had to deal with a hospital switchboard listens to this story in astonishment.

I told Mr Dent that I was a British doctor and I really loved Emergency Medicine and wanted to work in Melbourne, and I just thought that I would phone him on the off-chance that he might have a job. Then, to offer some kind of explanation for my slightly unorthodox approach to seeking employment, I finished by saying, 'Fortune favours the brave, and all that.'

Andrew Dent said that this was a great coincidence as he had, just that day, received funding for an overseas doctor and would I like to fax him my CV? The next day, a Friday, I faxed him my CV. On the Monday, I got a reply saying that the job was mine if I wanted it. I had certainly 'shown' everyone who was in the pub that night. That September I went to Melbourne.

I was twenty-eight. I wasn't in any way scared that I was travelling to the other side of the world, to a place where I only knew one person and had nowhere to live. The previous year had given me a kind of fearlessness that shocks me now when I look back on it.

Emergency Medicine had given me a sense of belonging and it began to do so again. However, I was very homesick. This came as a huge surprise to me. I had never experienced homesickness before. To begin with, I couldn't even figure out what the feeling was, and I still find it difficult to describe. It was a deep kind of ache, a feeling of loss that seemed to cut right into the core of my being, which would, out of nowhere, rise up and overwhelm me. What made it even more confusing was that I still had no sense of a place that I felt was home. So, I wasn't even grieving for a specific place. I was homesick for a home I didn't have. The quality of the light seemed to particularly affect me. It just seemed so bright and harsh, and I longed for the gloom and the smell of damp in the air.

Gradually, I began to settle down. I liked the people I worked with and started to make friends. I found somewhere to live, less than ten minutes from the hospital, and got on well with the people I shared with.

It was November. Spring was on its way; a magnificent time of year in Melbourne. By the end of the month, I was in a much better place, emotionally, but along came my old foe — Christmas. I was pretty confident that I would be able to hide from Christmas down-under. That's what everyone says, after all, about Christmas in the sun, it just doesn't feel like Christmas. Let me tell you, I could still feel it. Even though the Christmas trees and fairy lights were almost invisible in the bright sunlight, I could still pick up that festive glow. And with it came all the grief and loss I felt about my father, and that reignited my existential homesickness.

St Vincent's, or St V's, had originally been built to look after the poor Irish of Melbourne. Like all old institutions, it had its traditions. One of these was that, on Christmas morning, junior doctors would dress up and go round the wards, singing carols and handing out mince pies. People took this very seriously and would come in for it even if they weren't working.

Just before Christmas, one of the doctors stopped me. He said that people had been asking if I would be alone at Christmas, and, if so, would I like to join them for the carol singing?

I worked the nightshift on Christmas Eve, and then, on Christmas Day morning, I went over to the doctors' mess. On one side of the room were the costumes and on the other a table with beer, fizzy wine and an assortment of snacks. There was no messing about with the costumes; they were all from a hire shop. The choice was overwhelming, particularly after a night shift and a glass of fizzy wine, so I asked one of the others to pick something for me. She came back with the Dorothy dress from the Wizard of Oz.

Finally, the procession began. St Vincent's has a tower block and we started on the bottom and wound our way up. On the top floor we stood and sang *In the Bleak Midwinter* whilst I looked out the window at Melbourne shimmering in the heat below. In the ward, the tinsel twinkled in the sunlight and the Christmas tree in the corner was swallowed up by the glare from outside. And there, in the middle of it all, was me, feeling strange and lost, all dressed up as Dorothy. I was sleep-deprived, slightly drunk, and surrounded by superheroes, cartoon characters and a crew of anthropomorphic animals. Daffy Duck was having a conversation about blood results on the phone.

There are very few moments in life which are perfect, but this was one of them. The fantastical dream-like quality of the experience summed up how I felt better than anything else.

Toto, I have the feeling that we're not in Kansas, anymore.

## May 2022: Twins

After Zumba, I went to the supermarket. It was a warm day. The woman at the checkout smiled at me.

'I don't envy you in this heat,' she said, 'but not long now.'

It took me a few moments to register what she meant. Oh my God. How, how, how, after all the work I had done, how could I still look pregnant?

'When are you due?'

I couldn't say 'I'm not pregnant, I'm just fat.' Or even 'I'm not pregnant' and leave the 'I'm just fat' hanging there silently but still making its presence felt. And I couldn't joke about it because, frankly, I didn't feel like joking.

But I couldn't lie, either. Technically, I would make an excellent liar. I remember details, so I am less likely to be caught out. Also, I am a storyteller, and all stories contain a degree of lying; at the very least, a manipulation of the truth. But emotionally, I am not a good liar. I hate the idea that I'm deceiving people. So, I couldn't just say something like 'next week.'

Also, the part of me that pays attention to detail instantly recognised that to make up a due date was ridiculous. I go to the supermarket regularly; there was a good chance that she would be seeing me with my 'pregnancy' for some time; forever, at the rate that I was managing to lose weight.

And, somehow, creating a world in which I was pregnant was a line I didn't want to cross. My whole life seemed to be off-kilter. Standing in a supermarket pretending that I was pregnant would make it even more surreal. I didn't want to go there.

I gave a little laugh. Neither of us spoke. She looked at me, expectantly.

Unfortunately, I have never been very good with silences either.

'Not really,' I said. As an answer it had no logic, but I looked away in order to shut down the conversation.

'Oh, is it twins?' she asked.

I held myself together until I got back to my flat. Every time I went to the supermarket from now on, I would have to make sure that I avoided that checkout lady. But how? I could make sure that she was not serving at the queue I had chosen, but sometimes they swapped new staff in whilst you were waiting. And what if someone else asked the same question. Perhaps the safest thing would be to stick to the self-service checkouts. And I hated them for more than a few items. I would have to use a basket and not a trolley. It was so much more like hard work, but I couldn't bear being asked again if I was pregnant.

Why is this happening to me? I thought. Why? Why is the menopause being so cruel to me? Why can't I just be a normal kind of fat? A normal sort of fat that doesn't make me look pregnant. I would have given anything just to be normally fat.

I relived the humiliation. Part of me wanted to cry but I couldn't. Outside, someone was playing music. They kept playing the same song over and over again, and I lay on my bed with the same thoughts running through my head over and over again. It was as if I had somehow become trapped in a moment in time.

And not just in time; I felt trapped in my own body. There was something nightmarish about the whole scenario. It was as if my body was out of control. I no longer knew it. It was running rampant.

You are just going to have to diet harder, I told myself. But how? whispered the little voice in my head. What more can you possibly do? You can always do more, I answered.

You can increase your exercising, I told myself. Inside, I groaned. I was exhausted walking to and from work, and doing a Zumba class, with weights, every day. Maybe I needed to try other classes. Didn't people say that if you always did the same thing your body grew used to it? Maybe I had to shock it with different exercise. This idea was not appealing.

In that case, you will look pregnant forever, I told myself sternly. Don't you want to be able to use a normal checkout again? Anyway, you are probably exhausted because of all the excess weight you are carrying around. And everything else, like my job, I answered back.

Perhaps, the diet supplements might help. I felt a tiny bit of hope. But not much. I did not like relying on diet supplements to be my saviour.

You will just have to be patient, I added. But what was I going to do in the meantime? Buy maternity clothes? I had a sudden image of going into a shop to buy a maternity wardrobe and answering questions about the 'baby'. But perhaps there was something in the idea of buying new clothes, not maternity ones, just bigger ones. All my clothes felt tight. My tops were stretched over my ever-increasing belly. That probably wasn't helping.

Shopping is not the same when you hate how you look.

I logged onto M&S and selected six black tee shirts in a relaxed fit. I went up one size from normal. Then I remembered that I was now so big that someone had thought I was carrying twins. I went up two sizes from normal. As I finished the purchase, I did not get the usual little thrill.

It occurred to me that, as well as making me not want to go out for dinner, this was another thing my size was affecting. My weight was slowly robbing me of things that brought me joy. No wonder I was feeling so low.

Even work could no longer provide me with a safe haven. And I had always felt good there, or, at least, competent. But the current conditions made it impossible for me to feel as if I was doing a good job. In fact, I constantly felt that I was doing a bad job and that in turn was making me feel like a bad doctor.

I needed to do something to improve work, but so many of the things that were making it unbearable — the overcrowding, and the understaffing — were way beyond my sphere of influence. But, if I couldn't change those, I had to find some way of improving my relationship to work. I needed something like marriage guidance for me and Emergency Medicine.

## 1999-2000: Back Again

After that Christmas I settled down and started to love my job and to love Melbourne. My original contract had been for a year, but I extended it by six months and then a further six months. In the autumn of 1999, Andrew Dent told me that he would give me no more extensions.

'I know you'll think I'm being very cruel,' he said, 'but I'm doing this for you. You're a really good Emergency Medicine doctor so you can either stay here and join the training programme and I will support you, or go back home and train there.'

There were so many hoops to jump through to stay in Australia. And several of those hoops were exams. I would not only have to do exams as part of my training but also in order to gain full registration as an overseas doctor. And then there was the distance from my family.

I really did not know what to do. I chose to stay and then changed my mind; then I chose to stay again and then changed my mind back again. For someone as decisive as me, living in such indecision was hell.

I went to Tasmania with a friend and we took a boat trip round the harbour at Port Arthur. An icy wind cut through us, making our eyes water.

'If you keep on going,' the guide said, pointing out to the open sea, 'the next land mass you hit will be Antarctica.'

I had come as far as the sea could take me. Maybe it was a sign that I should go home.

It broke my heart to leave Melbourne. Sometimes people ask if I have ever thought of going back to visit. The truth is I'm scared to. I'm scared that if I did, I would just be filled up with regret. Also, I know that I wouldn't just be looking to revisit a place, but a time of my life that is gone forever.

Melbourne wasn't the only thing that I had fallen in love with; I had also fallen in love with Emergency Medicine. Right from the beginning, I had understood that one of the most important things is to keep things moving. Making a decision is key, and I understood that that is not the same thing as finding the 'correct' answer. Emergency Medicine is not about having to know a lot but more about being able to take what you do know and use it to decide what to do next. I loved the rhythm of seeing a patient, making a decision, seeing another patient and so on. I found it exhilarating.

I loved the excitement of it all, the unpredictability. Also, the specialty seemed to welcome everyone. Yes, there was a stereotypical Emergency Medicine doctor, a trauma-loving, adrenaline junkie. We all recognised and laughed at that ourselves. But that wasn't all. Emergency Medicine seemed to draw in all kinds of people with all sorts of quirks and eccentricities. Sometimes it felt like the pirate ship of the medical world.

People love the specialty because of its practical variety; you really do see everything. But for me, a natural storyteller, it is about the human drama. An emergency department is like a crucible of emotion, a great melting pot where everyone is turned up a few settings beyond normal. You see all aspects of human existence amplified: joy, sorrow, grief, guilt, fear, rage, hate, love, empathy, compassion, stoicism, humour, kindness, laughter, and stupidity. It's a register that moves from the sublime to the ridiculous and back again, taking in everything in between; it's a dizzy, dancing carnival, celebrating what it means to be human, swirling around you every day.

When you fall in love with Emergency Medicine, you can never imagine doing anything else. It would be like going back to black-and-white after living in technicolour. I'm not the only one that feels this way; time and again, I have heard colleagues talk about their passion for it. And passion is the right word. Those of us who love it, we keep on loving it, no matter what it does to us. We just can't help ourselves. We can't stop loving it, even though it is abusing us, burning us up, sucking us dry and spitting us out.

Despite this, we are often very forgiving. The problem isn't Emergency Medicine, we say; it's that we aren't able to do the job we love. And so, we hold on for grim death to keep the thing we love alive. We are fighting for the specialty every bit as much as we fight for our patients.

My love of Emergency Medicine meant that I was now, for the first time since graduating, fully committed and career-focused. In order to become a consultant, I needed to complete a training programme. The process has changed over the years, but the principles remain the same. You need to be accepted by interview onto an official training programme, on which there were — and still are — only a limited number of spaces.

Also, you were required to pass a series of postgraduate exams. I had — again — to address my *bête noir*, the dreaded MRCP Part 1, the exam I had kept on failing before I decided to go off and have a good time. Well, I'd had my good time, and MRCP Part 1 was still waiting. It consisted of thirty multiple choice questions. That might sound easy, but the wording was renowned for being incredibly tricky: for example, the difference between something *commonly* occurring in a certain condition, as opposed to *sometimes* occurring in it. MRCP Part 1 always focused on strange, rare conditions that no-one had ever heard of, let alone seen: conditions with names like tropical sprue or pseudomyxoma peritonei. Why on earth did they not ask about things that were relevant, rather than these rarities?

I wanted to be an Emergency Medicine physician. The likelihood of encountering any of these conditions was vanishingly slim. And I would never have to diagnose one of them. I would just need to recognise that someone was sick and refer them on for further investigation.

To add insult to injury, you had to pay to sit and — in my case — fail the exam. Part of me really believed that I would never pass. But now it was standing between me and something I wanted, rather than something I felt I should be doing. And so, my cast iron will and determination kicked in and, on my return from Australia, I immediately started studying for it.

I sat it in the autumn of that year. At the time I was working in Royal

United Hospital in Bath and living in doctors' accommodation. I was on a nightshift when I was told that the results would be out the next day. After my shift was over, I considered going to the mail room, to see if they had arrived, but decided instead to get a few hours' sleep.

People often say that waiting is the worst thing. I disagree. I don't mind waiting, particularly if it is for something that I might not want to know. It's not the waiting that is the problem for me; it's the finding out.

Finally, I made my way across to the mailroom. I had to wait in a queue, but I could see into the 'E' pigeonhole. There was one fat, brown envelope and a few white or coloured ones. There was a theory that if you had passed, you got a fat envelope as they sent you the application form for the next exam you were required to sit. If you failed, you got a thin envelope. I tried to stop myself hoping. I had always found hope a slippery thing that frequently lets you down. Disappointment after you had dared to hope always seemed so much harder to bear than straightforward disappointment.

When my time came, I was handed the fat envelope. I was shaking and sweating so much that I could hardly take it. I had thought that I would go back to my room to open it but, despite my hatred of finding out, now that I had it in my hands, I could wait no longer.

It simply said PASS. I had done it; I had defeated the MRCP Part 1.

I found it hard to settle after I came back from Australia. The old problem of feeling as if I didn't belong anywhere reared its head again. Or maybe I did feel as if I belonged somewhere; the problem was that it was Melbourne. When I told people that I had gone to Australia by myself, they said that I was brave. I always replied that, actually, it was braver coming back.

I got jobs in Bath and then Dublin but I yearned to be back in a big city. I got myself on a London training rotation in Emergency Medicine and when that was complete, I got a consultant post. I have been there ever since. There are lots of theories about how long it takes to become a Londoner. I read somewhere that you have to live there for twenty years. So, I guess I can say that I'm a Londoner now.

## June 2022: Double Whammy

My diet supplements arrived. I was desperate that they would work because they really did seem to be my last hope.

The comments just kept on coming. 'Are you expecting a baby?' and 'Oh, look at you, are congratulations in order?' That sort of thing.

It was a double whammy. Firstly, there was the shame of being so fat that people thought I was pregnant. Then when I had to tell them that I wasn't, they were so embarrassed by what they had said that I felt obliged to try and make them feel better. I feared their discomfort more than the horrible reminder about my size and shape. Sometimes, I tried to make little jokes. But there was something sour and curdled about them. I hated standing there trying to laugh about my size with other people.

I started to avoid people that I hadn't seen for a while. Scurrying along, always vigilant. If I saw anyone, I put my head down. Even when people didn't say anything, I became convinced that I could see them casting surreptitious glances towards my huge belly.

I knew that I needed to try and do more exercise, but it was hard. I was still so exhausted all the time. The thought of more classes was just too much for me. I was disappointed in myself and my lack of willpower.

When I was younger, I could push through anything and just keep going. I never had problems with doing more of anything: more work, more going out or more exercise. I could always reach inside myself and work harder. Now, I seemed to have lost that ability. It was yet another thing that made me no longer recognise myself.

I had requested a facilitated meeting to try and repair my relationship, and perhaps some of my colleagues' relationships, with the job. It was attended by those consultants who weren't off sick and some of our senior nurses and senior management. It was facilitated by members of the organisational development team. They encouraged us all to be open and honest and to say the things that are often difficult to say.

I know people can be cynical about events like this as they often don't generate any actions. But I believe that sometimes you need to spend time just talking about where you are and how you are feeling. If you are stuck in a situation, putting yourself under pressure to come up with a solution is really just a way of rushing to get out of it, without taking time to understand why you are there in the first place. You don't learn anything from the experience. We all know the old saying that insanity is doing the same thing and expecting a different result. Yet we often end up doing this. It is a lot easier to say than it is to recognise in ourselves.

As I said in the meeting, sometimes you just have to sit with the mess and the pain. We all have our own way of looking at problems, but this can give us a very narrow perspective. As problems are often viewed as threats, they can reignite all manner of memories and longstanding fears. It is helpful to hear how others view the situation. It's important to listen and to understand how everyone is feeling.

I'm a huge believer in Einstein's theory that you can't expect the thinking that caused the problem to solve the problem. In order to find a solution, you have to find a completely different way to look at a situation. Sometimes you can be stuck with faulty thinking and not even realise it.

During the meeting, I was able to express my concerns about the sickness rate amongst us as a group. I was sure that the high rate of injuries and illness was telling us something — and I thought that what it was telling us was that the job was becoming unsustainable.

Having had a chance to say how I felt, my feelings towards Emergency Medicine softened slightly — but only slightly.

## June 2022: Changing Shape

One day, I went to a coffee shop to get myself a drink. Afterwards, I used the bathroom. It had a harsh neon strip light: the kind that highlights every wrinkle and grey hair. Beside the sink was a full-length mirror.

On the rare occasions when I looked in the mirror, I was always clothed. But here, oddly, I was compelled to pull up my tee shirt and examine my naked stomach. I was shocked by what I saw. What hellish new development was this? Something even odder was happening to my shape. Whatever way I was gaining weight, there was an asymmetry to my abdomen. I bulged far more to my left than to my right. I studied myself in horrified fascination. I twisted and turned and looked at myself from various angles.

In the garish light, there was something distorted about my reflection; I felt as if I was in a hall of mirrors. When on earth had this happened? I thought back to my holiday at the end of February when I had studied myself in the hotel mirror. I hadn't looked like this then. Or had I? Surely, I would have noticed. How was this happening to me? Why was this happening to me? I just couldn't understand it. How could I be gaining weight with all my dieting? Maybe I wasn't gaining weight, I told myself, maybe I was just changing shape. It must be related to the menopause.

I was reminded of a PG Wodehouse description of a character as 'a tubby little chap who looked as if he had been poured into his clothes and had forgotten to say "when!"' That's how I looked.

I couldn't believe that this grotesque reflection was mine.

## 2016: The Wild West

I was from the generation of doctors expected just to get on with it. The long hours were to build up physical stamina; the constant being shouted at was to develop mental strength. Emergency Medicine requires a particular kind of toughness. Everyone shouts at you, both patients and doctors. Don't do Emergency Medicine if you want to be liked, for there will be days when absolutely nobody will like you.

One way of gaining popularity is to have something that others want. We refer patients to other specialties — giving them work, effectively — so you could say we have the opposite: something that nobody else wants. We are considered Jacks of all trades. We may not have the depth of knowledge that a specialist has, but we have a breadth of knowledge that they do not. The problem is that our professional conversations with other specialists tend to be on the subject in which they are the expert. That is precisely why we have chosen to speak to them. As a result, we are often remembered for what we do not know and, in some cases, what we have done wrong.

An emergency department is like the Wild West of any hospital: not quite in it but, instead, a frontier town. You have to have a certain kind of personality to want to work in that. And not just to deal with the shouting, but also the noise and the dirt; the unexpected, the uncertain. You never know what is about to walk in. You can be called away from a twisted ankle to deal with a fitting child; then to see a man who has chopped off his finger.

The more senior you are, the more tasks you are expected to do at once. Interruptions on interruptions on interruptions, like juggling fire, spinning plates and air traffic control all at the same time. No-one ever acknowledges that this mental gymnastics is a skill — as is making decision after decision. It's just another thing which we are expected to do and do quickly.

We also have to develop emotional resilience. Every day, we see a vast range of conditions, including truly horrific things: the son whose mother found him hanging from the banisters; the man who dropped dead in front of his children whilst out cycling in the park. Child deaths are particularly difficult: the toddler who accidentally hanged himself; the new-born baby killed when a car mounted the pavement the first time her mother took her out. All these burst into our days, brutally and unannounced.

We understand that this is just a shadow of what the experience is doing to the patient's loved ones. We are there in that awful time before the grief. We watch as a relative falls into the void, that period of incomprehension before the dreadful realisation of what the truth now is, of what life is now going to be for them. We sit with them in their grief, bearing witness.

Afterwards, we are expected to get back to work, to carry on and see the next patient. In the early days, you were told to take a few minutes out, get a cup of tea, go and sit in a tearoom or an office. You were encouraged to cry, if that's what you needed. You would sit there, and then you would get back out there. As I became more senior, the trauma began to be acknowledged, and we had debriefs, if we could. But in the end, you still had to see the next patient. And we all accepted this. This was the nature of the beast.

The patients that die are never forgotten. No one person remembers them all, but everybody remembers somebody. You carry them around inside you forever. Not just the sudden shocking deaths but the quiet, gentle ones too, and the people they leave behind, like the elderly person realising that the partner they have spent most of their life with is now gone.

Their stories become entwined with yours. Their ghosts live on inside you. There are some cases for which I remember the anniversary of their death; I silently acknowledge them each year. I think about their relatives. I am as haunted by them as I am by the patient that died.

Unpredictability was one of the things that drew me to Emergency

Medicine. How boring would work be if you knew what would happen each day? In Emergency Medicine, there was the thrill of the ambulance phone going off and learning that something dramatic was on its way. And, more rarely, but still a possibility, someone just appearing. On one memorable occasion, a man walked in carrying his own arm, ripped off by some agricultural machine. We lived for such moments.

The pace can go from quiet to busy in the blink of an eye. And you can never tell exactly when that eye is going to blink. However, it may not be as unpredictable as some might think. Most departments conform to a pattern of peaks and troughs. We know certain times of day when attendances rise, but there is always that unknown element which can throw the best-laid plans completely off-kilter. Working in an emergency department is like working at sea; a storm can blow up in a matter of minutes.

Anyone who wants to do Emergency Medicine has to be able to change gear quickly. People who like a steady pace always struggle. How you work is dictated by who, what and how many people are coming through the door. Emergency Medicine is a game of perpetual motion. If you stop the movement, everything will come crashing down.

When I first started, the job had a particular ebb and flow. There were times when you were required to be manic, and then the tide would go out and you would be left on a much quieter shore. Those quiet times were vital, for no-one could work at their fastest pace indefinitely. The down-times were when you bonded with your colleagues, got emotional support, and learned from sharing experiences. It was during these times that teams were built. The down-time was as vital as the hard work. Over the last decade, those down-times have all but disappeared. Any moment not spent improving productivity is viewed as a 'waste of time'.

I used to pride myself that there was no department so busy that I could not get it under control. I could always get things moving, get people sorted. I found it exhilarating and it was a major contributor to my job satisfaction.

For me, things started to fall apart in the winter of 2016. For the first time ever, I was regularly confronted by a department that I could not get under control. Now, I wasn't a superhero; I had obviously experienced bad shifts. But that winter, bad shifts became the norm. It was demoralising. I felt neither competent nor capable. I experienced this as a personal failing; I thought I'd lost my touch. This was happening nationally, so I knew, logically, that it was not to do with me. But what we feel and what we know are not necessarily the same. Feelings rarely accord with logic.

Languages are living things, always growing, and developing. Conflicts, for example, have added new words and phrases to our vocabulary. The First World War brought us 'cross the line'. In 2016, people who worked in Emergency Medicine coined a new phrase: 'Corridor Medicine': the act of seeing, treating, and looking after patients in the corridor. The problem was, in essence, a lack of beds: a lack of anywhere in the hospital to discharge patients to.

Having to care for patients in the corridor is dreadful for everyone: the patients, their relatives and the staff. It is a near intolerable situation. Corridor Medicine requires multiple adaptations to normal medicine. How do you take a good history in the noise of a public space? How do you keep what is said confidential? How do you examine patients whilst maintaining their dignity? How do you properly care for them, keep them warm and comfortable? What do you do if you suddenly need to resuscitate someone? And where do you find more space once the corridor is full? How do you do anything you're supposed to do for patients, both physically and emotionally, in a narrow thoroughfare that is not designed for this purpose? And how did any of this become acceptable?

Corridor Medicine is unremitting. It is exhausting and depressing. One of the nurses told me, close to tears, that some mornings she went home feeling a failure, not just as a nurse but also as a human being.

I was pushed beyond my limits one day in June. There were trolleys stacked everywhere and everyone was trying their best. It felt like the hottest day so far that year. I remember the medical registrar snapping, 'I can't possibly work in these conditions.' Sweat was dripping off his face.

The day wore on and the department seemed to heat up even further. Already frayed tempers reached breaking point and broke. Every task took longer, required more energy and was more frustrating than usual. The air seemed to condense and felt like a physical object to be battled through, as we tried to squeeze ourselves around the trolleys.

When I left, around midnight, the department was busy but no busier than usual. I returned at eight. The moment I walked in, I sensed that something was wrong. When you have worked in an emergency department for as long as I have, you can read the atmosphere like a book. And on this occasion, something palpable hung in the air.

The first person I saw was the registrar who had been the senior doctor in charge overnight. He was an excellent and experienced doctor. 'That was the worst night of my life,' was all he could say. The other doctors were huddled together, sweating, looking like they had just run a marathon or been at an all-night rave.

It was difficult for me to get to the bottom of why this shift had been so bad. After a nightshift, it's always hard striking the right balance between letting people talk, not interrogating them too much and allowing them to get home. It sounded bad — but just the kind of bad we were now experiencing on a regular basis: no beds, seeing patients in the corridor and large amounts of abuse.

The thing of note was the temperature of the department. Walking in from the freshness of the morning, I was immediately hit by it. It was hotter even than the previous day. It felt like being inside a greenhouse.

That's when I snapped. One of the best pieces of advice that I was given on becoming a consultant was never send an email when you are angry. That morning I broke it. I immediately fired off a full-scale rant about everything that was wrong. I finished with '...and finally, can someone please do something about the temperature of the department? It may seem a trivial matter, but it is not to those of us who have to work here. The department is unbearably hot. I am also conscious that some of the staff are pregnant, and others have just begun to fast for Ramadan.'

Perhaps because it was the only thing that anyone had a hope of fixing, everyone focused on the temperature. Several people appeared and agreed that it was, indeed, unbearably hot. They apologised and went to sort it out. Soon, I had an explanation. Apparently, there existed in the hospital a mechanism for blowing cool air into areas to control the temperature. As the weather was getting warmer, someone had decided to try and use it. Unfortunately, it had gone wrong, and had instead been blowing in hot air.

Some people may find it strange that I had never heard of this cooling mechanism, nor seen it in action, despite working there for eight years. Anyone who has ever worked for the NHS will not be surprised.

I was furious. I regaled anyone who would listen with the story. Most people just nodded and made their escape. Finally, someone said, 'Oh my God, that's awful, the poor patients, were they okay?' And that was it, that was the moment that everything changed for me. 'What about the poor staff?' I said. 'Why does nobody ever think about the staff?'

It was a question that I was to ask on many more occasions. What about the staff and their wellness and their experience? Surely, their experience at work is important too. Creating the correct environment for the staff should be as vital as creating the correct environment for the patients.

This was something that was to preoccupy — some may say obsess — me over the years that followed. It is something that I have probably thought about every day since and talked about to anyone who will listen.

## July 2022: A Touch of the Uncanny

One of the things that kept me going during May and June was the promise that staffing would be back to normal in July. Well, sort of normal. Most departments haven't had normal staffing for about a decade. And consultant staffing did improve as my colleagues returned from their sick leave. Take it easy, everyone said to them. Of course, they didn't: it is impossible to work in an emergency department and take things easy.

However, although the consultant rota had stabilised, there was now the problem of the junior doctor rota. July staffing is always tricky. Many junior doctors rotate in August, so there is always a scramble to use up leave. It's disingenuous to blame people for not taking their leave earlier. We are always busy and understaffed; there is never a good time to take it. It is inevitable that most people will not have used it by the end of their job. Anyway, leave wasn't the main problem; the main problem was sickness.

It was the hottest summer since 1976. Or perhaps even hotter, for we reached a forty-degree day. Extreme heat is as bad for your health as extreme cold, so we got even busier. It's also harder for the staff to work in the heat than the cold. Everyone was ill; we were up to seven doctors short. Writing the rota was like mapping the desert; it changed by the minute. You'd find cover for one shift and then someone else would phone in sick.

Working conditions felt toxic. The air seemed to be boiling. In the harsh sunlight, the city felt dystopian, and there was no let-up from the heat at night. Like everyone, I was having trouble sleeping.

I struggled to find something to wear each day. I had plenty of suitable clothes — one thing I was not short of was a hot weather wardrobe; it was the envy of some of my friends — but I could no longer fit into any of them. I had to struggle in my black jersey tee shirts and trousers.

I still wasn't losing weight, and the heat made it harder to exercise. I went for a walk on Hampstead Heath and felt so dreadful that when I got back home I had to lie down. And as soon as I lay down, I couldn't get up again. For the first time ever, I began to struggle with my Zumba classes.

Zumba had been another of those things that had kept me going through so many dark times. I generally looked forward to it; even on those rare occasions when I didn't feel up to it, I always felt better after a class. But now, even Zumba couldn't dispel my tiredness. I began to feel awful during the classes. I began to dread them. And this hurt me a lot. It felt like I had lost something else that I loved, due to my size. I hated my body for doing this to me. My fatness was robbing me of everything I loved.

One evening, I was convinced that I looked even bigger than I had that morning. I seemed to have gained weight during the day. Don't be stupid, I told myself. But I looked and looked and I was sure that I was bigger.

A couple of days later, a Saturday, I did a Zumba class which finished at eleven. I had certain things that I needed to do. Nothing big, just domestic chores and going to the supermarket. And I wanted to try and make myself go on a long walk. I made myself a cup of coffee and suddenly I felt drained. I was permanently exhausted, but this felt worse. I lay down on the sofa and closed my eyes. I really wanted to go back to bed, but I resisted. Going back to bed on a Saturday morning was a line that I didn't want to cross. So, I lay there, looking at the sky and watching occasional clouds drift past.

And time drifted past too, twelve o'clock, one o'clock, two o'clock; they all drifted by. Occasionally, I glanced at my phone: reading Twitter, nothing good, doom-scrolling. I slowly let go of my plans. The domestic chores would have to wait. I would not be going on a walk.

That only left the supermarket.

I wanted to buy some fruit and vegetables to make myself a salad for tea. That could wait as well. I could just have a boiled egg. But the thought of standing for the length of time it took to boil an egg was too much.

I needed milk, but I could just go to the corner shop. I was psyching myself up when I had a panic attack. I had never had a panic attack before, but suddenly I became breathless. I wasn't hyperventilating; I was just breathless. I felt as if I was gulping for air.

Why on earth was I having a panic attack? I was stressed at work, but I had been stressed at work for a long time. Everyone was stressed at work. Stressed was normal. I was also stressed about my weight, and exhausted by my failure to lose any.

Oh God, maybe what I was experiencing was due to my weight. Had I put on so much weight that I was starting to get breathless? I tried to think of medical conditions that my size could have led to. That is the problem with being a doctor and a patient. I suspect that you do neither well.

I tried to reassure myself that the episode was passing. Everything felt strange: the too-bright, overheated city; the hellish environment of work; my huge, bloated body. It was as if I had slipped into a parallel world. I felt scared, and not entirely sure what I was scared of. Nothing felt right; I couldn't explain it any more than that.

Stop it, I told myself; pull yourself together. You are being ridiculous. I lay with my eyes closed and slowly the breathlessness passed. Perhaps it had been an allergic reaction. I didn't normally get hay fever, but the hot air had that heavy, thundery feel. They were always talking about how bad the air quality was; maybe it was getting to me.

Finally, I felt normal. I made myself go to the supermarket. I didn't feel breathless carrying my bags. Perhaps I had imagined the whole thing.

Over the next couple of weeks, I had several more episodes, although nothing as dramatic as the first time. They lasted a couple of minutes and then passed. I wasn't even entirely sure if they were real or if I was imagining them. I had no other symptoms. Then, just as suddenly as they had started, they stopped and never came back. And I forgot all about them. Or maybe it was more that I chose not to remember them.

## 2016: Wicked Problems

The more I thought about what I could do to improve staff wellbeing, the more perplexed I was. The problems that the Emergency Department was facing seemed to be just the tip of an iceberg composed of government policy, finance, society, and the culture of the NHS, amongst other things. Although I didn't realise it, I was confronting what can be described as a 'wicked problem.' Wicked problems were defined by a design theorist and a city-planning professor in the 1970s, and they crop up on global, community and individual levels. They have a variety of features, but the key thing is that they are difficult or impossible to solve, because of their complex nature and their incomplete, contradictory and changing requirements.

Often, when we are faced with a problem, our inclination is to think of a solution and work back. With a wicked problem, all you can do is think of something that *might* make things better and try it. This may take you to a place where a previously unseen opportunity opens up, in what is called an emergent process. When I first read about this, it reminded me of something the writer EL Doctorow once said: 'Writing a novel is like driving a car at night. You can see only as far as your headlights, but you can make the whole trip that way.'

This more creative, emergent way of thinking — ie, let's just talk about this and see where it takes us — is much vaguer and riskier than a solution-based approach, particularly in an environment like the NHS. What if it takes us nowhere? What if it ends up being a total waste of time? These were risks that many were not willing to take. And it was not just time that people were scared of wasting, it was money too.

Given that many of our problems in the NHS — and also in life — are wicked, any idea is destined to fail if the desired outcome is a solution. Nevertheless, people prefer to keep looking for a silver bullet, a way of solving the situation, rather than accepting that it's a lifetime's work to make it better. This began to frustrate me more and more. You could be as innovative as you wanted, but only if you were able to guarantee that it would work.

I knew nothing about wicked problems. I was just angry at the situation and determined to do something about it.

My first idea was to hold a Schwartz Round. This concept originated in the USA in the 1990s, as the result of a legacy from a healthcare lawyer, Ken Schwartz, who had been diagnosed with lung cancer in his forties. He identified 'moments of exquisite compassion' that he had received from his caregivers, and recognised that staff needed support themselves. Schwartz Rounds, which have now spread to Canada, Australia, New Zealand and Ireland as well as the UK and the USA, have been shown to reduce anxiety and feelings of isolation in people who attend them. They are a way that organisations can show empathy towards their staff.

Schwartz Rounds last one hour, and keeping to time is very important. They always follow the same format. The rigidity and structure are important to help create a place of safety. Each round has two facilitators.

One of which is that we are not going to try to problem-solve. This is a big challenge for those of us who work in the NHS. We want to solve things, make it all better, sort it out and take away the pain. We don't want to accept that sometimes we can't and that we just have to sit with the mess.

Each round has a theme and begins with three or four panellists — clinical or non-clinical staff — talking about their experiences around this. They are encouraged to talk as if they were telling a story to family and friends. Then, one of the facilitators opens the round up. In truth, the panel is really just the warm-up act to encourage the audience to tell their stories.

This is how Schwartz Rounds work: they use the power and the magic of stories to unlock things that we have hidden away. All those things that we have carried around with us and, at times, been weighed down by, are given a voice and released into the room. Sometimes, it's sadness that is released; sometimes, it's deep-seated anger — the kind of fury that people bite back and bury inside themselves. It's surprising how many times people start or finish with the phrase 'I have never really told anyone this before'.

The facilitators gently stop any problem-solving. Even asking the panel too many questions, or trying to compliment or comfort them, is discouraged; there is always the temptation to hide from our own stories in the stories of others. In sharing stories, there is a feeling of connection, and a reassurance that we are not struggling on our own.

As a Schwartz Round facilitator, I am often asked to write about or say a few words about the process. This is a task I hate. To understand what they are really about, you need to experience one. The room is filled with an energy you can almost touch; a sense that, somehow, everything that we usually have surrounding us has been stripped away and suddenly we are just being with what is.

I decided that we would run a round just for the department, with myself and a colleague facilitating. Each round has a title, and I called this one 'The Winter of our Discontent'. In the planning stages, I learned an important lesson around introducing any initiative that involves staff, particularly in a department like the Emergency Department. The biggest problem is not coming up with something to do but finding a way to get staff released from their job — even just for an hour — in order to do it. This is why so many initiatives fail or never get off the ground.

The busier and more challenged the working conditions, the harder it becomes. Paradoxically, these are the times when it is needed the most. Unless something like a Schwartz Round is seen as an investment, as opposed to a luxury, change will never happen.

I managed to get enough people released by using a tactic that I was to use repeatedly over the following years. Sometimes it worked for me and sometimes it didn't. Basically, I went on and on and on about it. I may even have thrown a mini tantrum. Luckily, I work with great and supportive colleagues — and in this instance, I got my own way.

As per the format, the other facilitator and I met with the panel to hear their stories the day before. I sat there feeling overwhelming fury at what everyone was saying, along with sadness and despair that things had got to this stage.

In the round itself, when we opened it up, I heard more and more of the same stories. Everyone was feeling despair and hopelessness and not just at work; these emotions were also corroding their private lives. People felt that, for the sake of their own health, they could no longer go on; they didn't want to leave but they felt that they were being given no choice.

But, although some people did leave, many just kept coming into work. It was something that I was to see time and again, through the next few winters, and the pandemic, and its aftermath. We kept trying to do our jobs as best we could, whilst all around us the goalposts kept shifting and things got harder, and we all got more and more tired. And I think this commitment was because, at its heart, we were doing a job we genuinely loved and believed in.

The job we fell in love with has all-but-disappeared in amongst everything else, like the horizon in a storm, but we keep on coming back. Why? Who knows? Maybe many of us can't stop hoping that one day the storm will eventually pass and, just like the horizon, we'll be able to see the job we love clearly again.

## August 2022: Trapped

I quite like August. It feels like the start of a new school year. It's doctor change-over time and the new doctors who arrive in the department bring both excitement and optimism.

Staffing improved, but I was still exhausted; I complained to my equally exhausted colleagues all the time. I began to think about reducing my hours.

'Emergency Medicine is a young woman's game,' I said, frequently. 'It's not the same when you are over fifty and menopausal — you can't work the way you used to.'

For the first time ever, I felt I couldn't cope with the hours. Previously, I had easily done twelve-hour shift after twelve-hour shift. Now I was finding work not unlike the way I now found having a hangover: I needed a longer and longer recovery time. Once I was able to have just seven or eight hours between shifts and still show up, bright-eyed and ready to go. Sure, I might have joked about needing my coffee, but that was no different from any morning. And I didn't really need the coffee, I just liked it.

Worse even than the hours was the uncertainty. Approximately once a week we were on call: we did a clinical shift from three in the afternoon until eleven thirty at night. Then we were available by phone for advice and would come back in, if need be. The problem was that with the staffing issues and general business, we often could not leave on time and had to stay on until we felt that it was safe to go.

I began to worry about having to work beyond midnight. I feared I might collapse if I had to work that late. I knew I was being over-dramatic, but I began to have a feeling of terror whenever I thought about having to work longer. The fear and dread simmered inside me and I felt furious with the NHS and its unreasonable expectations.

As my anger intensified, I thought of everything that I had given to my job. All those years of hard work, all those years of going the extra mile. I had sacrificed my youth for it and what was I getting in return? Just the expectation that I would continue to make sacrifices. My extra efforts had been normalised. Finally, a day would come when I had nothing left to give. I suspected that, at that point, I would be spat out and forgotten about.

Sometimes, I would say, 'When I'm retired or dead, whichever comes first...' And that was no joke. Emergency Medicine doctors are the ones most likely to die before retirement. We might worry about our pensions, but how many of us wouldn't get the chance to draw them? That would be the final irony. It made me think of my own father. He, too, had worried about his pension, only to die at fifty-eight. Was the same fate awaiting me?

All these dark thoughts sucked me down like quicksand. They took me to a place from which I struggled to escape. One of the reasons that I had become interested in staff wellness was that I feared my dark sense of humour was becoming too cynical. I recognised that cynicism is a mere hop, skip and jump away from bitterness. I never wanted to be bitter, but that was what I was becoming. I was disillusioned with my job; I was disillusioned with the NHS; I was disillusioned with everything. And, oddly, this was harder to deal with than the fear and the dread. Naively, I had always believed in what I had done; it was what had kept me going. I had believed that I was doing some good. Now, I wasn't so sure.

I had to spend most of my weekends that August catching up on admin. I was incensed that I had to give up my spare time to do it. Looking back, it had always been that way. Right from the beginning, that was what made you appear dedicated: that you were prepared to go the extra mile — invariably for free and in your own time. It was the culture.

But, as well as being incensed, I was also relieved. That's another thing about work; it's a very good place to hide from the rest of your life. You can avoid lots of other things and look virtuous whilst you're doing it.

I was getting pregnancy comments all the time, from random strangers as well as from people I knew. One Sunday afternoon, I was walking home after a particularly busy shift. I hadn't eaten much and it was hot. I felt dizzy. A woman approached, riding her bike on the pavement. It had one of those carts attached, with two children in it. The cart swung towards me and I had to use what little energy I had to jump out of the way.

'Don't worry,' I said, when she apologised, and then I made the mistake of making eye contact and smiling at her.

'When's your baby due?' she asked.

'I'm not pregnant.'

I didn't just say the words: I spat them out at her. I'll never forget her expression. She looked shocked and turned away. I was shocked too, shocked at the rage I heard in my voice. Not just rage but also frustration and pain. Everything I was going through came out in those three words. It was the only time I answered that question as I truly felt; the only time I didn't try to evade it or laugh it off or try to make the asker feel okay.

The other thing I heard in my voice was incredulity. I was incredulous that, despite everything, I still looked pregnant. And incredulous as to why someone would ask a complete stranger a question about their body.

I have never been pregnant, but I know that pregnant women often comment on how, as soon as their pregnancy shows, other people feel that their body is now public property. I could really identify with that. I didn't feel that my body belonged to me anymore. I had lost all control of it.

I simply couldn't tolerate any more exchanges like this and so I hid away in my flat as much as I could. All my confidence ebbed away. I was like a hollow shell of myself. Except I wasn't or, at least, that was not how I looked. I looked like an overstuffed cushion. I felt lost in my own body.

Occasionally, I would remember the person I used to be. I wanted to cry, but I couldn't quite get there. I was rigid with fear that the person I used to be was gone forever, and I wasn't going to be able to get her back. This was my new normal. Trapped in this body and stuck in this flat.

## 2016: Joy and Dancing

In early 2016, the pressure started to ease. It became possible to believe that, perhaps, things were improving and that the last months had been some kind of anomaly. But, deep down, I feared they would return. I could see that many of the issues that had come up were still there. People felt undervalued and unheard. There was a disconnect between what was expected of us and what we were able to achieve. I couldn't let go of the idea that something was gravely wrong in the NHS as it didn't seem to care about the wellness of its own staff.

Who was I talking about when I said the NHS didn't seem to care about its staff? I didn't realise it, but what I was beginning to think about was that elusive thing we refer to as culture. Culture is one of those words that is frequently used, but it's not always clear what people actually mean by it.

I continued to think about it. Unbidden thoughts would creep into my head as I was walking home from work, or on the tube.

One of the main things that had got me through that never-ending winter was Zumba. Zumba is a group exercise class, based around Latin American and African dance moves. I had started it in 2011. As part of my never-ending battle with my weight, I have been a gym-goer on and off for most of my adult life. Initially I wasn't enthusiastic about the idea of dance. I was the wrong shape and had no sense of rhythm. I had no coordination, and I could never figure out the steps in time. Unfortunately, however, Zumba had replaced several classes that I was doing at a time that suited me.

I stopped going to the gym altogether for a few weeks. Finally, I gave myself a stern talking-to. Okay, I said, go and try Zumba. If you hate it, you can find another gym. So, one dismal Thursday night, I found myself waiting to go into the class. The place was packed. I had never seen it so busy and there was a buzz in the air. I was bemused, and also quite anxious. It's okay, I told myself. Just stand at the back, do the class. Who cares if you do it wrong? Then, another little voice added, 'Who knows? You might even surprise yourself and find out that you actually enjoy it.' It's safe to say that I was, indeed, about to give myself one of the biggest surprises of my life.

The first track was a salsa. Obviously, I had heard salsa music before, but I suddenly understood something that had totally passed me by. This was music to be danced to. It was a kind of euphoria that called for me to be part of it, and how could I not want to be part of it? How could I not want to dance? I didn't want to do anything but dance.

I could feel the beat vibrating through the floor. If it had been a cartoon, silvery wraiths would have risen up and wrapped themselves around my feet and then made their way to my heart. It was as if my whole body had been possessed, like the girl in the fairy tale of the red shoes.

Now, when I said I hated dancing, that wasn't strictly true. I adored indie music and indie clubs, so, yes, I had experienced the joy of wanting to dance and never stop. But that was at about 2am to Pulp singing *Common People*, with alcohol involved, not on a Thursday teatime in the gym.

I completely forgot that this was exercise. This was a joy. I wanted it never to end. I just wanted to be there, in that room, dancing forever. When it ended, everyone was smiling. I left the gym filled with a crazy, wild energy and had to walk home, rather than getting the bus, in order to dispel it. Inside my head, my brain was playing a Latin American soundtrack. And so started my obsession.

I looked around a class, one Saturday, and it was full of different types of women: all ages, shapes, and sizes. It was a bright morning, and the room was full of sunlight. There was a woman in front of me who was much larger than I was. I could not take my eyes of her and the way she moved to the music. She was magnificent. She had such a joy about her. I thought of all those classes where I had tried to force my body to conform to a different shape, to mould myself into something that I wasn't. This was the first time I had ever exercised and not felt like I was fighting with my body.

Dancing, like many other things, requires a certain mindset. Overthink it and you're screwed; let your mind wander and you're screwed. It requires that particular balance point where you are all focus and very little thought. This is the state that some people call 'flow'. It's the point where you are so absorbed in a task that you are no longer worrying about the future or fretting about the past. You are totally in the present. For that time, you are safe from all the thoughts that hold so much worry, unhappiness, and pain. For a brief period, you get a break and it's glorious.

The other thing that had kept me going during that difficult winter of 2015/16 was my writing group. I had loved writing as a teenager and had always wanted to write a book. But, like many things, that ambition had been forgotten as I grew older. However, several years earlier, I had had a difficult and painful time in my personal life, and so, one very dark January weekend — dark in both my mood and the weather — I had remembered my old desire to write, and joined a weekly writing group. The focus was not on producing a finished piece of work, but on developing a regular creative practice and having fun with it.

During the sessions, we would engage in a variety of writing exercises but the aim of them all was the same: to get us to write without stopping and, more importantly, without thinking. I found the idea challenging and, quite frankly, ridiculous. How could you do anything without thinking?

Maybe I could write without thinking, but it would be nonsense. What I wrote when I was thinking would obviously be superior. We had to read out what we had written, and I wanted to read out something good. This wasn't to show off; I felt that if I did anything, it ought to be good. All my life I had always tried to turn in the best work that I could, so it seemed alien to produce something that was nonsense. Nonsense equates to rubbish.

But, by just doing this every Monday night I learned, in time, that you *can* write without thinking. In fact, the less you think, the more you write. Maybe some of it *is* nonsense, but it's less nonsense than you might imagine. When I sifted through what I had written, I found things that amazed me.

I realised that I had limited control over what I wrote. What wants to be heard will always find a way to make itself heard. Often, after I had written a piece, I would realise that it had been about something that had been on my mind without my paying much attention to it. I would only discover what was important, and what I should be writing about, after I had written it.

Just as dancing requires the mind to be in the balance-point of focus and absence of thought, creativity requires a similar state. And so, a bit like dancing, it was another thing that let my mind settle in the present for a while. The process itself was very soothing, even if what it generated was surprising; even if, at times, it took me somewhere I didn't want to go. Often the things that you don't want to face are better faced in the end. No matter how dreadful, they are much worse when they lurk in the darkness.

Writing calmed me. After I had been attending every Monday for about two years, I had to stop for six weeks, due to another commitment. During this time, I felt out of sorts and jittery. I couldn't, initially, put my finger on what was wrong. Then I realised that I missed writing.

Dancing and writing had kept me going through that long, dark winter. I recognised it was important that every day I did something that brought me joy. It didn't solve the problems or make them go away — often, I would walk to Zumba class or writing group feeling anxious or tired or fed up, and by the time I got home I was already feeling anxious, tired, or fed up again — but at least the class had changed something for a short time. It had given me a break and that was immensely beneficial, like glimpsing the sun through the clouds.

## August 2022: Disconnected

I was sick in August. Nothing serious, just diarrhoea and vomiting. Lots of people had it, both staff and patients. I had begun to feel strange and gone to the bathroom. It was another of those bright, neon-lit bathrooms. Yet again, I was shocked by the appearance of my abdomen. For a moment, I thought that I resembled someone with a bowel obstruction.

I felt so unwell that I had to go home from work and, shortly afterwards, I began to throw up. As I lay in bed, vomiting violently, I began to wonder if I did have a bowel obstruction. At what point should I seek medical help? I told myself not to be ridiculous; it was just that I felt so sick.

The next day, although I still felt delicate, I decided I would keep my appointment at the hairdresser's. My huge belly remained unchanged. I hadn't expected a day's vomiting to cause me to lose weight, but in the past, in a similar position, I would have felt a little smaller, if only due to the amount of fluid that I had lost. But my belly was as large and as firm as ever. I might have been disappointed, but, in a way, I wasn't surprised. My belly seemed determined to hang in there no matter what I did.

After my appointment, I made my way to the tube. It was a hot day, and I really did not feel great. There was a huge crowd of people on the platform. A young woman beat me to the only empty seat but, seeing my large belly, she immediately jumped up and offered the seat to me. I was about to decline but I accepted the kindness. If you don't sit down, you might faint, I told myself. A woman with a young son smiled sympathetically, but I tried not to make eye contact; I did not want her to ask about the baby.

When the tube eventually arrived, it was packed. The little boy sat on one of the 'baby on board' seats but she shooed him away and beckoned to me. I really felt that, as she had observed the previous encounter, I couldn't refuse. Anyway, I felt seriously unwell and was grateful. I was horrified that I was now basically pretending to be pregnant in order to get a seat on the tube, and horrified that, owing to my bizarre shape, I could.

Odd as it sounds, I am not entirely sure when my chest disappeared. I have no idea if it went gradually or quickly. I was so focused on my large belly that I didn't really notice anywhere else. I had always had big breasts. Like many of my friends in a similar position, I would complain about this, frequently, to my smaller-breasted friends. They, in turn, would complain to me about their shape. Is that not often the pattern of female conversation?

But, like my smaller waist, my larger breasts had always been part of what made me, so it came as a bit of a shock when, one day, I realised that they seemed to have vanished. Above my 'bump' I was completely flat. I wondered if it was because my belly was so large that it was making my chest look smaller. Could my belly be compressing my breasts in some way? No, I concluded, they were definitely shrunken.

It was as if they had withered away. More cruel behaviour from the menopause, no doubt. They resembled two deflated balloons resting on the huge swell of my abdomen. I may have longed for a flat chest when I was young but now that I had one, I wanted my old one back.

My bras were now all far too big. They hung on me, sagging and underfilled. When had this happened? It was hard to believe that my breasts had just disappeared overnight, but how had I not noticed earlier? My body and I were so disconnected that I had no idea what it was up to half the time. I really didn't understand it. We were like a couple who had stopped loving each other a long time ago and really should think about getting divorced.

## 2016: Forum Theatre

Whilst I was using dancing and writing to get through 2016, one of my colleagues took up running. She had been going home, feeling miserable and having a glass of wine, which wasn't making her feel any better.

'I just realised that this is all shit,' she said, 'but the situation isn't going to change any time soon, so I had to look and see what *I* could change.'

This really interested me because I was just about to take part in a departmental initiative using Forum Theatre. I had first heard of this a few years earlier on a course at the Central School of Speech and Drama, which used methods taught in acting to improve communication in doctors.

Forum Theatre, devised in Brazil in the 1950s by Augusto Boal, sees theatre not just as a form of entertainment, but as a tool to drive social change. The process consists of a play where an identifiable protagonist faces a series of seemingly insoluble problems, which are either harming them or preventing them from leading a fulfilling life. A Forum Theatre piece always ends badly for the protagonist, who will be defeated by the problems that they are facing. Following the performance, a member of the cast, the Joker, who has not appeared in the drama, takes to the stage to facilitate a discussion with the audience. The Joker encourages the audience to think about where things went wrong for the protagonist, and asks: could they have changed their behaviour to get a better outcome?

After the discussion, the play is re-run. Second time around, the audience is encouraged to shout 'Stop!' at any point where they think that the protagonist would be better served by behaving differently. Whoever shouts is then invited on stage to try out their approach to see if it works.

Obviously, there are rules. The audience can only ever replace the lead character and change his or her behaviour; they can't replace anyone else. They also have to be faithful to the reality of the play; they can't suddenly say that the lead character has inherited a lot of money and is now a millionaire. The other actors are committed to their roles and behaviour and will resist changing. But sometimes, depending on what the main character does, they are persuaded to change.

The process works particularly well when members of a specific community work with practitioners to develop a piece which is relevant to them, and the problems they face. The performance offers an opportunity to think about these together and share their knowledge.

Forum Theatre seemed to be an exciting way of exploring the problems we encountered and never solved in the Emergency Department: problems that were a complicated interplay of the system, the personalities involved and the conflicting priorities. It took all the different facets and the way they interacted with each other into consideration. This was much more realistic than the often simplistic way we approached things.

Forum Theatre recognised that often it could not *solve* a situation for its leading protagonist, but it could make things better. It could find ways of helping them exist in a system that appeared to be working against them.

I loved using drama to recreate our problems and challenges. It was able to bring them to life and highlight their complexity in a way that discussing them did not. It made them real — so real, at times, that you stopped playing and were back in the noise and chaos of the department.

Subsequently, I have been involved in a variety of Forum Theatre projects which we were able to introduce to the department. One was with Cardboard Citizens, a professional theatre company, and others were with master's students in Applied Theatre Studies from Central School of Speech and Drama. In each of the projects, we ran a series of workshops with some of the team. We created a scene which we performed as a Forum Theatre piece to an audience on the last day. As in all creative pursuits, it wasn't just the end point which was important, but also the process by which we reached it. The workshops gave participants the chance to discuss their experiences; they allowed everyone to reflect deeply and gave them time to process what had happened. They offered opportunities to recalibrate and rejuvenate. People seemed refreshed afterwards.

Initially, many people were sceptical that they could create and then act in a piece of drama. But they were all capable. The level of talent that came to light in every project was astonishing and uplifting to watch. People surprised themselves, discovering abilities they were unaware they had.

The workshops were very playful and involved a lot of games. As in my writing group, fun and playfulness were inextricably linked to creativity. Game-playing was very much part of the process; it was not some kind of add-on before everyone got on with the serious work of creating something. The games were the work of creating something.

I had experience of this from a few years previously, when I had been going through the very unhappy and painful time that had first led me to writing. To try and figure out what I needed to do in order to feel happy, I had booked myself onto a laughter yoga course.

I set off full of good intentions. After introductions, we started off by playing a game, then another and then another. The more we played, the angrier I began to feel. Time was ticking on, and I wanted to get down to the serious business of tackling happiness. Not running round a room with a whole lot of other adults as if we were children.

When I think back, I often wonder what I thought we should be doing in the pursuit of happiness. I suspect that I thought we should be having a long, philosophical conversation about it, something intellectual, where we might share our experiences and maybe learn some kind of theory. That would have been very much my comfort zone. Playing games certainly wasn't. I felt silly and self-conscious. As the morning wore on, I had to come to terms with the horrible idea that the games weren't something we were going to do before we got down to the important stuff of the session. The games were the session. There was going to be no important stuff.

I even thought about running away at lunchtime. But there was no opportunity because we all ate together, so I gritted my teeth and headed back for the afternoon. Only a few hours to go, I told myself. I sat there hating everything and everybody. Beneath my anger, I could sense other things: discomfort, unease, a feeling of being disconnected. And, beyond that, there was all my misery, all the stuff that I had come to deal with.

Then, I got it. Something just clicked. This is the only way I can explain it. We had moved onto improvisation games and perhaps that had ignited the performer in me. I did something and everyone laughed. So maybe I required a degree of approval or even praise.

I could analyse that afternoon for a long time and come up with more and more insights about myself. Underneath all the apparent silliness, the games go very deep and frequently unearth stuff. But they are not an intellectual exercise. They are not there to be discussed or analysed or even thought about. Not at the time, anyway. They are there to be played. They require activity and they require concentration. Like all healthy activities, they take you from that place in your head, full of worries and anxieties about the past and future, and they force you into the present. And, as they are fun, the present is a place full of laughter.

None of this occurred to me at the time. I was just playing the game and laughing. My attitude changed towards the others too. I was no longer an outsider; I was part of the same group. I found myself liking them and perhaps I liked myself a bit more, too. Of course, the games didn't solve or fix any of the stuff that I was trying to deal with. Those feelings returned soon enough; it would be a while before I was able to move beyond them. But they did lighten up that day.

There are games for everything. Games to energise you and games to calm you down. Games designed to get you to focus, and games designed to get you to connect and work as a team. Games to explore communication, body language and tone of voice. In theatre, they are used as warm-up exercises. They start the process of improvisation and they are used to develop the piece. They are there to turn individuals into an ensemble.

When I started Forum Theatre workshops with the team from the Emergency Department, I noticed some people would always be dubious initially — although, to be fair, no-one was as hostile as I had been. But within a short time, everyone would be relaxed and laughing. At the end, the feedback would always be about how much everyone had enjoyed the games. People commented how great it was just to have the opportunity to play or be playful: something that they had not done for so long. Everyone would walk out of the room laughing, lit up, exhilarated even.

In these projects, the team involved came up with scenarios based on their experiences of working in the department. We created quite complex scenes, to explore seemingly intractable problems. These generally involved situations where the system, combined with the behaviour of others, would end up leaving staff feeling defeated. We would spend time developing all the characters, so we would look at reasons why patients, their relatives and other staff members would act the way they did. This was a useful exercise in allowing the team to consider what was driving the behaviour in others: fear, perhaps, or anxiety, or their own work stresses. Most people involved said that the project helped them be more empathetic.

These scenes were very real. They represented recognisable dilemmas. So, when the audience thought about the question 'What could the lead character have done differently?', they were really asking themselves, 'When I am in this situation, what can I do differently?'

But did Forum Theatre really work? That was the perpetual question — sometimes asked, and sometimes implied. And here is the conundrum: how can you really tell if something works? The feedback after every Forum Theatre project, from both participants and audience, was always excellent. However, that sort of feedback really only measures how much participants have 'enjoyed' the experience.

Of course, this is the same for any educational session. After a talk on how to manage heart failure, the feedback will focus on the speaker's delivery. No-one measures if it actually changes management of heart failure. That seems to be irrelevant. The very nature of the talk means it is addressing an important issue, and that is enough to make it a worthwhile investment. But with more creative projects, there is always anxiety about whether it has 'really worked'. Has it just been a waste of time?

The majority of complaints we receive are not about poor medical management but poor communication. Similarly, the biggest cause of medical errors is related to poor communication. These are the dynamics that Forum Theatre is excellent at exploring.

But the question remains: can I ever prove that it works? In these resource-strapped times, can I really justify taking people away from their job for the time required? Can I ever prove that, in a hospital environment, giving people the opportunity to immerse themselves in a creative project is anything more than an extravagance?

Forum Theatre also poses another challenging question: how much can you expect any individual to change in order to cope in a dysfunctional system? Or, put another way, what should you turn your attention to: individuals or the system? As staff wellness became increasingly under discussion, this was an argument that I was to come across frequently.

The system undoubtedly needs to change, but I recognise that this is difficult and will take time. So, whilst that is happening, our staff need to be supported, not simply to prop up a failing system but so that we are doing the best we can for them. As healthcare professionals, we manage chronic disease whilst still searching for a cure.

Boal later realised the limitations of the process: there is only so much the protagonist can change by changing his/her own behaviour. Frequently, a change in the law or the system is needed. When he served as a *Vereador* (the Brazilian equivalent of a city councillor) in Rio, he developed a new kind of theatre called Legislative Theatre, the aim of which was to open a dialogue between individuals and institutions. In this instance, the drama focused on laws and their effects, and explored what laws needed to be changed or introduced to support communities and individuals. During his time as a *Vereador*, thirteen new laws were created, based on this learning.

## September 2022: Imprisoned

I was still tired; work was still busy and despite my best efforts, my belly was still huge. I was constantly aware of it. It seemed to take up so much physical space and mental space. It was the first thing that I thought of when I woke up, and the last thing I thought of before I went to sleep.

Every morning, I would run my hands across it and then look at it under the covers. It rose up like some sort of great dome. I would scrutinise myself in the mirror, hoping that it looked smaller. But it never did. It was still massive, with that odd asymmetry to it, bulging out more to the left than the right, and my withered, shrunken breasts lying on top of it. I hated it.

In September, the weather grew colder and so I had another clothing dilemma. My winter wardrobe was usually more forgiving than my summer one. But I couldn't find anything that fitted. Everything looked terrible on me, pulled and distorted over my massive stomach. In the end, I just continued wearing my old, faithful tee shirts with a long-sleeved vest underneath. They had become a uniform of sorts.

I stopped doing Zumba. It broke my heart, but I was just too tired to continue. During the classes, I felt sick and physically uncomfortable. I had never thought of Zumba as exercise; I did it because I loved it. But now, I just couldn't do it anymore. Every time I did it, I was reminded that it once brought me so much pleasure. Also, if I'm being honest, it was something that I had felt good at and now I couldn't bear being bad at it. Maybe that's how I felt about work as well.

Of course, I didn't admit to myself that I was giving it up forever. I just told myself that I was having a break from it. I was going to be away quite a bit in October, so I told myself that I would restart in November. But even as I had the thought, I knew it had a hollow ring to it: this was yet another thing that I loved that would slip away from me, due to my age, the menopause and my size. But it was my shape that was the thing that really bothered me, more even than my size. I was just such an odd shape.

In work, I now avoided going out into the main part of the hospital as much as I could. I dreaded meeting anyone I knew. Even if they didn't say anything, I imagined that they were looking at me, speculating. I imagined people talking about me, discussing it amongst themselves.

Patients had started questioning me too, which made me fearful of going to see them. And as that was fundamentally my job, that made me dread work all the more. Out on the street, I kept my head down. Complete strangers could pop up from anywhere and accost me. I was always vigilant, always wary; the only place where I felt truly safe was in my flat.

The irony that I was menopausal but was constantly being thought of as pregnant did not escape me. Sometimes, I tried to reassure myself that at least I must still look quite young. Other times, I was grateful that I had no regrets about never having had children. It was bad enough as it was, being asked about when my baby was due, but if childlessness had been an existing sorrow, then the situation would have been unbearable.

There was something else about my shape that bothered me: it just didn't feel right. It felt unnatural. It really unsettled me being like this. Why did I look pregnant? I had never heard of this happening to anyone else. At least, I had never heard of it happening to anyone due to weight gain.

My body was like a disobedient child and I had let it behave like this. But I had tried so hard. Nobody could have tried harder, I told myself, but it just didn't seem to be enough. Another thing that was just like work.

I began to fear my own body, for I no longer felt in control of it. I was now its prisoner.

## 2016-2017: Survivorship Bias

Throughout 2016, staff wellness was constantly on my mind, but it would be another year before I could do anything else about it.

Getting doctors to take breaks has always been problematic. We talk about how important it is, but the system does not support it, and, to be honest, the culture and mindset of many doctors does not help. There exists in medicine the view that taking breaks or leaving on time is a sign of weakness. Soldiering on and going above and beyond is seen as a virtue.

One reason for this is survivorship bias. If a system is challenging, only certain people will survive it. They will progress through the system, and, in time, some will assume positions of power, including being able to influence the design of the system. However — and this is the critical thing — as they survived it, they are less likely to see the obstacles that prevented others from progressing and less likely to make the necessary changes. The opinions of people who had to drop out are rarely sought. Often, being able to survive in a particular system is seen as a sign of strength, and an inability to survive as a sign of weakness. Surviving becomes a pre-requisite of the job. The flaw is attributed to the individual and not the system.

We now recognise that not taking breaks is a safety issue. It's not safe for patients or staff for staff to work long stretches without a break, so in recent years organisations have become keen to promote the idea that breaks are important. As a result, it began to be mentioned at new doctor inductions, which occur each time the doctors rotate: two or three times a year.

For many years, it was my responsibility to give the 'break' talk. My talk was infamous. It was, in my opinion, a towering work of black humour and cynicism and very tongue-in-cheek. Some people 'got this' and found it hilarious; others didn't and found it terrifying.

I began by saying, 'This is a bleak and unremitting job.' Then I talked about 'Things that I can guarantee', one of which was 'You will all cry.'

However, it was removed from the induction. This, I hasten to add, was nothing to do with the quality of the talk. It was felt that 'breaks' could not be given a whole time slot and so they were mentioned at the end of the 'Welcome to the Department' talk. I didn't really mind. Humorous as I thought my spiel was, I had come to the conclusion that it was a waste of time. It never actually achieved anything. Some of the audience may have laughed, but it didn't get them to take their breaks. Similarly, those who found it and/or me terrifying didn't take their breaks either.

The reasons people didn't take breaks were a lot more complicated than not being told they needed to. I felt that I was oversimplifying something that was more complex than I was acknowledging. Then the inevitable happened, and some of the juniors complained that they never got breaks. An action plan was required. Point one was a talk about breaks in induction. I was reinstated. Point two was posters. Could I perhaps make some?

'Make some posters of what?' I asked.

'Posters reminding people to take their breaks,' was the answer. To say I was unenthusiastic is an understatement. People did not forgo their breaks because they forgot, and so seeing a poster reminding them was not going to change anything.

I duly gave my break talk at the next induction and, no doubt, amused some people and frightened others, though my heart was no longer in it. But as for making a poster — that was pushed to the back of my mind where I quickly forgot all about it. Or, at least, I thought I did.

Where do good ideas come from? I think that they come from our subconscious, that great and uncharted part of the brain. Just because we don't know what it's up to doesn't mean that it isn't busy. Our subconscious is constantly trying to talk to us via things like dreams and bright ideas that just appear. The problem is that we often miss what it is trying to say, as it's drowned out by all the other noise around, including the thinking mind. But sometimes it gets through.

This is my explanation for why, one evening as I was walking home, the phrase 'If you don't take a break, you will end up broken,' popped vividly into my head.

At once, I thought that it sounded like an advertising slogan, and this was instantly followed by the idea that I could put it on the posters. I had totally forgotten about them. Mercifully, so had everyone else.

What sort of graphics would go with that slogan? I asked myself. Isn't that just typical of how your mind works? When I had been told to do something, I had resisted. Now that it was off everyone's radar, I was on board. I had a brainwave. I could use an image of an X-ray of a broken hip. I could have a whole series of posters, all with commonly missed fractures. I could make it into a competition.

Now that the idea of Take a Break had captured my imagination, I couldn't stop thinking about it. At first it was just an abstract concept, but the more I thought about it the more I realised that it was achievable.

I went in on my day off and made the posters. And yes, I could see the irony in that. I was encouraged when others started to comment on what a good idea it was. I knew that putting up posters wasn't enough; I had to create a buzz around them. I started by talking about them all the time and promoted the quiz. I recruited some of the junior doctors to act as champions. I imagined it as my version of a public health campaign.

The big question is: did it work? The answer depends on what you judge as success. Did it solve the problem of doctors not taking their breaks? Of course, it didn't. But, by the end, people were taking more of their breaks. So, you could argue that it made things better.

I have continued to run the Take a Break campaign ever since. Have I solved the problem now? Are all of the doctors taking all of their breaks all of the time? The answer is still no, but I hope that I have continued to make things better.

It has taught me a lot. Interestingly, despite my love of it, the initial Take a Break poster campaign and quiz was of limited use in encouraging people to take their breaks. The answer to 'what is the difference between a quiz and a test?' is a prize, and I didn't have enough money to fund a sufficiently desirable prize to encourage people to participate.

What was important, though, was the fact that I had done something. I had named it and talked about it and brought it out into the open. And by doing this, I had changed something. It may have been a little change, but it was still a change. Perhaps the first step in changing any culture is to name the change that needs to be made.

No matter how compelling and persuasive I tried to make my induction talk, it was never enough to persuade people to take their breaks. Not taking breaks was so ingrained in the culture that one talk was not sufficient to change things. I started sending regular emails to juniors stressing the importance of their breaks. I was careful how I phrased them too, so they didn't sound like a rebuke.

What did work was good role modelling. If juniors saw seniors taking breaks, they were themselves more inclined to take them. What also worked was feeling part of a team where the culture was to remind each other about the importance of breaks. The biggest reason for not taking breaks was always related to busyness and, specifically, busyness caused by understaffing. When the department had the optimal number of doctors, people were all more likely to take their breaks.

The other thing that Take a Break changed was me. It ignited something in me. I hadn't just thought about staff wellness or talked about it, I had actually done something, however small. It struck me again how the wellness of staff was never really considered. It was not so much the elephant in the room but a dog that never barked.

## October 2022: Confusion

At the beginning of October, I had an online meeting with a colleague, and she commented that I looked like I had lost weight. I felt a little thrill of pleasure until I realised that she couldn't see my belly, which was still as huge as ever. But I looked at my face on the screen and it did look a little thinner. I always have had a relatively thin face and so it was the last place I needed to lose weight. Maybe it was a sign that my dieting was beginning to work, and my belly would be next. Afterwards, I tried to look at it in the tiny mirror in my office, hopeful that it, too, might look smaller. Maybe it did, fractionally, but I couldn't really say.

October brought with it both a blessing and a curse. On the positive side, I was off work for most of it and also for the beginning of November. I was delighted and relieved to be away from the department. I had not designed things this way; they had just happened. I had planned a holiday and then had been asked to speak about staff wellness at two different conferences, one after the other.

It occurred to me that this might be something that was contributing to my tiredness. In order to get a large block of time off, I had had to work for a large block without a holiday. This was the sort of thing you can do when you are young, but which seemed rather foolish at my age.

The first event was the Royal College of Emergency Medicine autumn conference. I was excited about that. Firstly, it was an opportunity to speak about something that I felt passionately about. Secondly, I'm a performer at heart and I love an audience. Thirdly, I was excited about speaking because the conference was to be held in Belfast. I had begun to think about home a lot. This was unusual for me as I had spent most of my life not thinking about it very much at all. The last time that I had properly lived at home was when I was at school. Back then, all I had wanted to do was leave. I had never imagined coming back. But now, much to my surprise, I found myself longing to be there. I started to joke about giving up my job, selling my flat and moving back to Portrush.

I had learned a long time ago that often the things I am most serious about start off as jokes. The more I joked about it, the more tempting it became. I was finding it difficult to cope with everything. My job was becoming harder and so was living in London. I was staying in my flat most of the time, anyway; I was terrified of going out and being ambushed by questions. I might as well go home and stay in. It would be cheaper.

I couldn't help but think that my adolescent self would be very disappointed with me. All I had wanted to do, then, was to go off and have an adventure. But now, I felt that those years had passed, and I just wanted a gentler way of life. Everything seemed so much of a fight, and I was just too tired to struggle anymore. I began to say that I was five or six bad shifts away from resigning. And the way that work was, most shifts were bad. I had definitely fallen out of love with Emergency Medicine.

When my flight landed on a grey, drizzly day in Belfast, I let out a great sigh of relief and felt that I could breathe again. I had planned to stay for a few days in Portrush with my family before and after the conference. I was in no hurry to get back to London.

I went down for the conference on the day before. I checked into my hotel and, as I was waiting for the lift, I caught a glimpse of my reflection. I looked massive. Actually, I didn't; I looked heavily pregnant. My reflection was distorted and fragmented in the mirrored tiles.

As soon as I went into my room, I looked in the mirror. After a period of intense scrutiny during the summer I had returned to the other extreme and had avoided looking at myself over the last few weeks.

As I stared at my reflection, my appearance was very confusing to me. I did look like I had lost weight but only in certain places: places where I didn't really need to lose it, such as across my shoulders and my arms. I now looked like a very slim, pregnant woman.

I thought that if it wasn't for my belly, I might look quite slender. But I couldn't ignore my belly: it was huge. There was something about it that didn't even look real. I felt as if I was looking at a caricature of myself. Except it wasn't a caricature, it was me; I really did look like this. I still had the left-sided asymmetry, but I couldn't decide if it was different or not. I tried to remember what it had looked like previously, but it was like looking at a landscape and trying to decide if it had altered in some way.

There was something about the size and shape of it that made it three-dimensional. It looked different viewed from different angles. It almost didn't seem part of me. Worse, it looked bigger than ever. But surely that was impossible? With all that dieting, my belly couldn't still be getting bigger? Also, I told myself, your dieting must be working in some ways: look at your shoulders and arms. My shoulders and arms were — something I never thought I would say about myself — verging on the point of being too thin. Perhaps my belly only looked bigger as everywhere else was getting smaller. It was some kind of optical illusion. If I just kept on dieting as I was, then surely my belly would catch up eventually.

Then another terrible thought hit me: a much more pressing concern. I was about to stand up and speak in public looking like this. I was horrified. Why had this not occurred to me earlier? Perhaps I was in some kind of denial about everything. I had tried to control the full horror of my appearance by hiding away — like a teenager concealing a pregnancy, I couldn't help thinking. I had a dirty, guilty secret that I was determined to hide from the world. Perhaps I believed that if I could hide for long enough, that I would be able to solve the problem, but that hadn't worked either. All my best efforts had been for nothing — although, not entirely nothing, I reminded myself, glancing at my skinny arms.

I had been looking forward to the conference so much, and I couldn't bear the idea of it being spoiled by my appearance. I just hadn't let myself think about it. I was so sick of this. And so tired.

I was reminded of the time just after my father had died, when it had not occurred to me to dread Christmas until Christmas was upon me. Why the hell did I not think about this problem earlier?

It wasn't just wasn't the talk that was the issue, I realised. One aspect of any conference is the opportunity to network. That meant there was a whole network of people out there to wonder if I was expecting. I felt myself begin to panic.

First things first, I told myself, and went to try on the dress I had chosen to wear for my speech. It was another stretchy old friend. Mercifully, it fitted. If anything, it was a bit loose around my shoulders and flattened chest. Unmercifully, this accentuated my huge abdomen. Well, it would just have to do. Actually, in the end it didn't have to. I just wore my usual uniform of a large tee shirt over vest and black trousers.

The conference was unremarkable, at least from the perspective of people asking me if I was pregnant. And I saw quite a few people I hadn't seen for some time. I was always anxious though, and wary. I kept my distance, both physically and mentally. It was as if I had erected a barrier around myself to discourage conversation. It was the antithesis of who I was as a person and it made me sad to be like that. But what else could I do, apart from resolve to diet harder and lose the weight so that people stopped asking me when the baby was due?

At times, it seemed an almost comical predicament, and I had moments where I wondered how my life had come to this. Why was my body doing this to me? I was having to cut myself off from everyone because of my appearance. I was trying so hard to lose the weight, but nothing seemed to be happening; at least, not to my belly, where it needed to happen.

When I got back to London I was off again, almost immediately, to the second conference, in Berlin. Obviously, I was exhausted. So exhausted, in fact, that I forgot to take my Kindle. I only discovered this on the tube. I'm one of those people who doesn't mind long periods of waiting or travelling as long as I have something to read. Since I was a teenager, I have always had a book or a Kindle with me. I have left my keys or purse behind more frequently than my book. I couldn't believe I had left home without it.

The first thing I did when I arrived at the airport was to buy myself a novel, but I was already feeling a bit chaotic and out of sorts when I met the friend I was travelling with.

'You've lost weight,' he said.

I smiled in surprise. It wasn't what I had expected. It was true that I was losing weight from my face, arms and shoulders, but I didn't think that was enough to get a 'you're losing weight' comment. My belly was still huge, and I felt it overshadowed the rest of me. But I supposed it was positive that some kind of weight loss was now noticeable.

There was something about the way that he said it, though, that didn't sound quite right.

'Are you okay?' he asked.

'Of course I'm okay,' I replied and then added my usual, 'just very tired.'

We sat in silence for a few moments. Then he said, 'I'm just saying this as your friend, but do you not think you should get checked out?'

I was confused. I hadn't lost that much weight.

'Have you had any other symptoms?'

What was he talking about? Of course I hadn't had any symptoms. For the briefest of moments, the panicky breathlessness from the summer passed through my mind.

'I'm fine,' I repeated. 'Just tired,' and I began to read my new book, shutting down the conversation.

Normally, I was having to shut down conversations about pregnancy; now, I was having to shut down a conversation about… well, I wasn't sure what, exactly. It was all very confusing, and I was too tired to try and make sense of things. So, I just shoved it to the edge of my consciousness where it was easier to ignore.

## 2017-2018: Fun Theory

After the Take a Break initiative, in 2017, I began to think about how I could change the culture. I started to research how to run a successful advertising campaign, which is how I came across Fun Theory. Fun Theory was devised by Volkswagen, when they were looking for a way to persuade people that they could be more environmentally conscious whilst still being car drivers.

Their research suggested that people are more likely to change their behaviour if fun is involved. One of the most famous examples comes from Odenplan Underground Station in Stockholm. The aim was to encourage people to use the stairs rather than the escalator, so they turned the stairs into a giant piano that played music. Stair usage increased by 66%.

I already knew that a playful environment was vital for creativity. However, I felt that making things 'fun' was frowned upon. Playfulness was often conflated with childishness, and 'fun' things carried less gravitas. I sensed an unspoken rule that things which were important should also be serious. To be taken seriously, you had to be serious. Putting the word 'theory' after 'fun' seemed to legitimise it in some way. Also, there was now the all-important evidence to show that fun worked.

There was hardly any information about staff wellness back in 2017. The little that I could find identified it as an issue that needed addressing but provided no advice on how to go about that.

I wanted to make staff wellness a 'thing.' I felt that the more that I talked about it, the harder it would be to ignore. I formed a wellness steering group which consisted of me, our service manager, and our practice development nurse. In time, I started calling myself the Staff Wellness lead. This was a title purely made up by me but, in conceiving it, I created the role.

I learned an important lesson here. The more formal titles we had, and the more people that were involved, the more credibility it gave and the more 'real' the concept became. It was also much easier to get things done when there was more than just me.

As I've said, one of the challenges of trying to introduce anything is getting staff released to attend. This problem has dogged me continually. Initially, I wrote a couple of wellness talks. I decided to deliver them at lunchtime, but no-one was ever able to come. I spent several weeks trying to think of how to get people released until the penny dropped. I couldn't.

Departments all start getting busy around eleven o'clock. That's one problem. Also, people don't want to give up their lunch break for a talk. And there is an irony in expecting anyone to give up a lunch break to listen to a talk on wellness.

I was looking at this all wrong. Instead of asking myself, 'How can I get people released at lunchtime?', I needed to ask myself, 'How I can find a way to give these talks?' By reframing the question, I found an answer.

We provide ten minutes of teaching in the department every morning. Anyone can attend as long as they are not dealing with an emergency. Some of the slots were vacant and I decided to take them. Also, I wanted to do something more than just give talks. So many things about the job were making people feel unwell. I couldn't change those, but I wanted to do something, however small, to make people's days a little better. Like the idea for Take a Break, the idea of playing warm-up games just popped into my head one day. Initially, it seemed a bit mad, but I had seen the positive effect that the games had had on the workshop participants. They cheered everyone up, energised people and encouraged everyone to work as a team.

When I suggested this to the other members of the steering group, I did so slightly tongue-in-cheek, but they loved it. It was agreed that the practice development nurse would facilitate the games. On the first morning, I sent everyone off with her and I stayed out in the main department.

I was so anxious that I was sweating and felt sick. What if something happened? This was a completely irrational fear. But that's the thing about something new, it's always a risk. The ten minutes seemed like hours. Finally, everyone came running back out. I immediately felt the shift in energy.

'That's really woken me up,' someone said.

Everyone was smiling and laughing. One of the doctors later told me that they had initially thought, 'What the hell is going on?' but then had really enjoyed themselves.

I started to try and do one session every week and called the initiative Pop-Up Wellness. I discovered that someone in the Trust was an artist, and he came and did a brief talk and got everyone drawing. This was something else that I was to learn: there were many talented people around who were excited to share their skills. Other events included silk painting (from one of our paediatricians) and origami (from one of the pharmacists). Another of the paediatric consultants was a member of the Magic Circle. He came a few times and did a magic show for the team, which was very popular.

I hadn't started with a fixed plan; I was making things up as I went along, but something was beginning to take shape. Fun and creativity worked like meditation or mindfulness, as they focused the mind on the present.

Laughter has been shown to have multiple health benefits. It reduces blood pressure; it increases beneficial hormones such as serotonin and oxytocin whilst reducing more harmful ones such as cortisol; it is good for reducing stress. The evidence around laughing in groups is also interesting. People tend to laugh more easily and for longer if they are in a group than if they are alone. Laughter bonds people who laugh together.

This resonates with my experience of what happened when we played games. When it worked well, it was exhilarating. There was a warmth in the room, and you could feel the connection between everyone.

There was no way of predicting this. I just had to go with the energy that people brought. But even on days when things felt muted, the energy in the room was always different at the end. The games had moved people to a different place, and it always felt to me to be a better one. It really is true that if you are stressed or angry about something it helps if you can take your mind off it, even for just ten minutes. It may not solve the problem, but it can change your relationship with it.

I became aware of my own resistance to playing the games. I would make all sorts of excuses to myself to get out of it, but I learned to ignore these. No matter how I felt before the games, I always felt better after them. I recognised that, on occasions, I wanted to stay angry or annoyed about something because deep down I didn't want to let it go. I either couldn't or wouldn't imagine that I could be in a better place. But I always forced myself to play and invariably felt better for it.

Creativity is also shown to be beneficial for wellbeing. In 2019, the World Health Organisation published a meta-analysis of all the studies that had looked at the effect of creativity on both mental and physical wellbeing. It revealed a positive link. In one study, doing just ten minutes of something creative every day was shown to result in increased feelings of positivity.

I can easily believe this. I have seen the focus and concentration people show when absorbed in a creative task; the simple joy when they see their creations come to life. And somehow, in revealing this side of themselves, it encourages people to open up about all sorts of other things too. I began to see the people I worked with in a whole new light; tiny little things, but I experienced so many moments of connection with the team.

Of course, the big question, as always, was did it really work? I had excellent feedback but, in the long run, did it make any real difference?

After one of the sessions, one of our nurses told me that he thought it was very good that I was making an effort, but, ultimately, he felt that it was a waste of time. He was leaving nursing, he said. He didn't want to; it was all he had ever wanted to do, and he loved being a nurse. But he couldn't continue in the current conditions. It was too stressful, he could no longer do the job that he wanted, and he was struggling to survive on the salary.

I went back to my office deflated. It was heart-breaking; the NHS was full of enthusiastic, dedicated people and we were driving them away. And he was right: what good was it, really, getting people to play a few games? How could that possibly reverse the effects of working in poor, under-resourced, underpaid conditions? I had no power to change the things that needed changing.

I thought about it. I might not have solved the problem, but at least I had created a space where people felt open and able to talk about how they really felt. Even if I didn't like what they were saying, it was better that I had given them an opportunity to say it. And it was better that I had given myself the opportunity to listen to them. I had not fixed anything, but perhaps, I had made it fractionally better. And even if I hadn't made it better, I had at least made it different.

In February and March, we had the opportunity to run nine Wellness Days. We came up with a programme of events based around fun and creativity.

Everyone loved the days, and I loved running them. I got to know the team that I worked with better in those nine days than I had done in all my time working with them. There was nothing sophisticated about it. We had allowed the team one day away from normal work to spend time with each other having fun. It was all about connection and getting the team together. In the end, we had one hundred and ten staff members attend.

Once again, feedback, using a validated wellness score, was excellent. Even more illuminating were the comments: 'wonderful day'; 'a meaningful investment in staff'; 'so lovely to spend time with colleagues in this way'; 'got to know my work colleagues better and made me feel more appreciated'. Touchingly, some people just wrote 'thank you for doing this for us'.

'But did it really work?' I was asked. Did it reduce sickness rates, for example? I found it unlikely that one day could do that but, in the end, I looked at sickness rates that April and compared them to the previous year. They were down by thirty-three percent. Of course, I can't say that this was to do with the Wellness Days. It wasn't, however, due to a mild winter. Early 2018 was the time of Aussie flu and the Beast from the East.

## October 2022: Something New

At the end of October, I was a facilitator on a communication course. I was part of the team, along with airline cabin crew, who had developed this.

I loved running the course. It gave me the opportunity to do everything that I felt passionate about: talking about communication, facilitating really great conversations, using drama and other innovative techniques for learning, and connecting with people. There were occasions when people really opened up, and we had some deeply moving moments where attendees felt comfortable talking truthfully about their experiences and were willing to be vulnerable within the group. I always observed that, in any format, when this happens, people in the room really connect to both the person and what they are saying to create a truly powerful experience. It was important to me to be able to do something that I believed in.

This was a stark contrast to my job which, I realised, I had stopped believing in. I no longer felt that I was doing any good — just firefighting and trying to hold things together. I normally ended a communication course feeling as if I had done well, whereas I left a day at work feeling utterly defeated and as if I had done a poor job.

The only problem with the course was that it meant that another area of my life which I truly cherished was being affected by the 'pregnancy problem'. I was constantly on show and so there was no hiding my huge, bloated belly. Also, as we encouraged connection and invited people to open up, there was a very real danger that someone might innocently say the words I was constantly dreading: 'When's the baby due, then?'

As I was doing in all other areas of life, I tried to reduce the likelihood of this by controlling my interactions with others. I avoided mixing during the coffee breaks. When I wasn't facilitating, I put up a protective shield up to deter anyone from getting too close and asking questions. Even if no-one said anything about me being pregnant, I knew that that's what people in the audience were assuming. And I hated that too.

It had been a good course. Everyone had been really interactive and there had been lots of laughter and lots of serious conversations too. As we were leaving, I let my guard down a little and one of the delegates asked the inevitable question. I gave my usual tight little smile and made my usual tight little joke.

'I'm not pregnant,' I said. 'Quite the opposite. I'm menopausal.'

The woman who, through the course, had shown that she was a lovely, warm, kind person, was horrified. I felt dreadful, really dreadful. She gave me a little hug and apologised.

Then she said, 'But you've had everything checked out, haven't you? You're alright?'

'Yes, yes, I'm fine,' I replied.

'Here's me telling a doctor that they should get themselves checked out,' she said.

I smiled but, as I did, it hit me: I'd never got this checked out; never even thought about it. Perhaps people might be surprised at that. They might think that, as a doctor, that would be one of the first things I would have done. But, maybe, as a doctor, I didn't think that I needed to. I didn't think that there was anything wrong with me. I had just put on weight that I couldn't lose. I didn't feel unwell. I felt uncomfortable at times, but that was due to my size. I didn't have any other symptoms and I wasn't going to see a doctor because I'd put on weight.

All the way home, her words kept popping into my head. I tried to push them away. But it was proving difficult. The place where I stuffed my unwanted thoughts was full, like a cupboard where you shove your junk. The door would no longer shut, and things kept on falling out.

I remembered what my friend had said at the airport. I hadn't really thought about it since. But he, too, was telling me I needed to get checked out. I didn't want to get checked out. I felt a coldness pass through me, as if I had accidentally swallowed an ice cube. What if there was something wrong with me? I had a hunch that if there was, it wouldn't be good. I couldn't tell if this was the doctor me or the person me.

I felt as if I was standing on the edge of panic, about to fall in. I pulled myself back. Stop it, I told myself, firmly. There is nothing wrong with you, nothing at all. Look at how many hours you are able to work. Surely if there was something wrong with you, you wouldn't be able to do that.

'But you're so tired,' said the little voice inside my head.

Everyone is tired, I told myself; everyone is exhausted.

'Maybe you could see your GP about the weight?' said the little voice.

It was tempting. I was desperate. I had tried everything. For a moment, I fully admitted to myself how much this was affecting me. The idea of someone helping me felt almost overwhelming. Then I remembered what the doctor had said when I was a child. I couldn't bear hearing that again.

'What? That would be more humiliating than everyone thinking that you are pregnant?' prodded the little voice. 'Anyway, things have moved on a little since the seventies. There are lots of treatments for obesity. Maybe you could have an injection.'

I thought about it. Perhaps I would qualify for Ozempic.

When I got home, I was very tired. Too tired to eat anything. But that was fine by me. All the better for my diet.

I went to bed early but lay awake. I was having to work very hard to stop myself thinking. Little thoughts kept escaping. They were like sheep that I had to herd up and put back into their pen. It was like the opposite of counting them to go to sleep. All those little moments of humiliation.

But there was something new there too. My shame had some company inside my head. There was fear in there as well.

## 2019: Two Steps Forward, One Step Back

I felt elated after running the Wellness Days: elated that we had done them and elated by the response. What I needed to do was to start to promote the work. I gave presentations. I joined Twitter, now X, and began tweeting about it. I became a prolific tweeter, so it is comical to remember that, at the time, I had no idea how Twitter worked. I had to get one of the other doctors to give me a tutorial.

The year started on a high. I went to Australia to a family wedding and then onto a creative writing retreat in India. Whilst there, I discovered that an article about the Wellness Days, which I had submitted to *The Guardian*, several months earlier, had been published. I received lots of positive feedback. I returned to work brimming with enthusiasm and ideas.

Unfortunately, due to a combination of factors, things did not work out quite the way I thought they would.

Jo, the practice development nurse, and Nicola, the manager, got other jobs and left. So now it was just me rather than a steering group. Trying to do anything on your own is so much harder, especially when there is no authority behind what you are doing. If I had been trying to do something established or mandated, it would have been easier.

Secondly, there was the issue of money. We had been able to use existing funds to run the previous Wellness Days, but now I had to get funds for future events. I tried numerous avenues but none of them got me anywhere. I told myself that every time I tried and failed was good practice for the next time I had to try to get money. I got a lot of practice.

However, money wasn't exactly the issue. It hadn't been a commitment to the process that had allowed us to run the previous Wellness Days, rather a desire to use up money that we already had, so that we wouldn't lose it. Now that there was no fear of losing money, there was no push to plan further events. Added to this, we were — as ever — experiencing staff shortages and so it was harder to release people to do anything, let alone a full Wellness Day.

This is a problem that is still plaguing hospitals up and down the country. It's a vicious circle. People are leaving the NHS. This puts more pressure on remaining staff, but it becomes harder to release them for anything as they have to work constantly to try and plug the gaps. This ultimately burns them out and/or drives them away... which puts even more pressure on remaining staff, and so on.

It's all very well having a long-term view, and ideas about how to improve the situation, but when you are struggling every day just to keep things going, it's hard to make change happen. In amongst everything else, it was hard to find a space for something as unproven and novel as the Wellness Days, particularly given they were based on fun and creativity. They seemed the ultimate in frivolity.

I became very despondent and disillusioned. One of my friends, who worked in organisational development, gave me some very good advice. She pointed out that I needed to stop trying to fight the system and just wait and see what opportunities came my way.

So that's what I did. I let go of any new, grand ideas, at least for the meantime, and went back to what I did have — ten minutes once a week — and waited to see what would happen.

One initiative that we managed to introduce was taking tea together. The idea came from one of our senior nurses, who told us that he had once worked in a department that served afternoon tea every day. Every day seemed too ambitious, but a couple of colleagues and I decided that we would give it a go one afternoon. We bought some cakes and biscuits and at three o'clock we got everyone who was available to have a cup of tea. It went down very well.

It grew into a weekly tradition: every Thursday at three o'clock. We called it *Tea at Three*. As time went on, it became more and more extravagant. It turned out we had a talented collection of bakers only too happy to show off their skills.

We tried to invite as many people as we could: doctors from other specialties, porters, security and anyone from the ambulance service who was around. One of the most touching moments came when one of our porters, originally from Bulgaria, asked if he could provide the food one week. He wanted to do a Bulgarian *Tea at Three*. He said that he was in awe of all of us in the department and what we did for others, and wanted to find some way of expressing this.

*Tea at Three* was not popular with everyone. Such initiatives often come under fire in the great debate of what we should focus on: the system or the individual. Treats are all very well, but people argue that they distract from the real issues. We need to provide good working conditions, proper rest areas, lockers, free parking, twenty-four-hour access to hot food. Not to mention proper pay, flexible rotas, and adequate staffing.

I agree. I have never proposed that *Tea at Three* is a substitute for these; that, somehow, a piece of cake is an adequate replacement for everything else that needed — and still needs — to change. But I continued to believe that it was important to do something whilst we waited for any big improvements to occur. Also, *Tea at Three* was more than just cake. It went back again to the idea of building community. One of the oldest ways known to build meaningful connections is to break bread together. Food, and feeding people, is a well-established way of showing love. In the challenging times in which we were working, it was one of the few ways I could think of showing love to my colleagues and my team.

I tried a lot of other things in 2019, some of which worked and some of which didn't. Thanks to *The Guardian* article, and also to my prolific tweeting, a few people became interested in what I was doing. I was interviewed by workplace culture expert Bruce Daisley, for his podcast *Eat, Sleep, Work, Repeat,* which is all about building positive workplace culture. Then I was contacted by a publisher who had read my *Guardian* article, to see if I could write a book; in the end, that did not come to anything.

That was the pattern of the whole year. Sometimes it felt like two steps forward, one step back. But I got better at dealing with it as time went on, and became philosophical when things didn't work out.

I started to be invited to speak at other hospitals about staff wellness, and, towards the end of the year, at a few conferences. One, held in November, was run by NHS England, and was all about culture change. I remember a feeling of excitement in the air, and a notion that there was a real desire to change the culture and a definite will to do so — and a sense that it was possible.

At the beginning of January 2020, I was invited to speak at a conference based around creativity and wellness in health care professionals, held in Margate at the Turner Contemporary gallery. It was a beautiful location and a beautiful day. The room was full of people passionate about staff wellness and passionate about creativity. In the late afternoon, we had a break, and everyone went outside to watch the sunset. Turner had chosen to live and paint in Margate as he said it had the best skies in Europe. Looking out over the sea, as the sun set, it was easy to see why. The whole thing felt magical and I left feeling happy, and optimistic about the future.

A few days later, I received an email from someone that I had met there. She finished by saying that she hoped that my work was okay, and that we weren't being affected too much by this new, terrible-sounding virus. I often think back to that email. It was one of those moments where life seems cinematic, like when someone in a film says that they are going on a sea voyage and then the camera pans in on their ticket to reveal the words *HMS Titanic.*

## March 2020: Border Control

On 10 March, 2020, the UK government allowed the Cheltenham Festival to take place, despite growing concerns around the novel coronavirus. Say what you like about the government — I frequently do — but on this subject, I am a little reticent, because on that day I made my own rash decision, and flew to Essaouira, Morocco. Essaouira is one of my favourite places in the world. I've been there several times, on creative writing retreats run by my friend, Claire, and I had been looking forward to this one for ages.

Of course, I was fully aware of the coronavirus, as we were still calling it back then. We were starting to see cases in the hospital and we were onto the second or even third management protocol by then. I had seen the footage from China and, more recently, Italy.

But I was really in need of a holiday. I had been under the weather for ages. I was having stomach pains and they just wouldn't go away. There was no way I was going to cancel. Everything will have blown over by the time I get home, I told myself. The old joke is that denial isn't just a river in Africa — and for me, it turned out to be a town in Morocco. Denial was something that I was, in time, to realise that I had quite a talent for.

When we arrived, Essaouira was as beautiful as usual. On the surface, it was easy to forget about the rest of the world. But, despite my best efforts, the rest of the world kept intruding. People kept on mentioning coronavirus, at breakfast or in the souk. It felt like an ambush. I didn't want to talk about it, and I didn't want to think about it.

On the evening of Sunday, 15 March, I went to meet up with the others to go out for dinner. We always met in Claire's room and had a gin and tonic together. As I walked in, she handed me a glass and said, 'Sit down.'

She had learned via social media that, due to coronavirus, Morocco had shut its borders. She had little other information. The hotel owners were in the same position. We spent the next three days trying to find a way to get out. It always surprises me now that it was only three days because, cliché that it is, it felt like a whole lot longer.

However, every day, Claire made us write.

'We have come to write and that's what we'll do,' she said.

Are you out of your mind? I thought, the first time she said it. How can you possibly expect us to write in these conditions? And anyway, there are so many other things we should be thinking about; we don't have the time to write.

Then it struck me: like what? What other things had we got to be thinking about? We were waiting for information. I was unwilling to write, because it would interfere with my worrying and fretting. Or maybe I felt that the worrying and fretting was much more powerful than my ability to write. What I learned was that it wasn't. It took a bit longer for my mind to settle into the writing but, miraculously, it did, for a few hours, at least, and I could feel the benefits — so much so, that when I got home, I continued to make time to write and have done so practically every day since.

Essaouira shut down. The hammams and the restaurants closed, as did some of the shops. We wandered through those that were still open and bought things we didn't really want — as much for the shopkeepers as for ourselves. We could sense their fear as well as our own. Everyone was brittle. We were all holding ourselves together. By then, 'ourselves' was just a very thin shell stretched over fear.

We were told, by the Consul, to wait for information about rescue flights. When we didn't hear anything after a couple of days, we decided that we would go to Marrakech Airport, to see if we could find a flight home. Shortly after we made this decision, however, our airline advised us that there were spaces on a flight from Agadir the next day. We booked ourselves on.

As we drove out of Essaouira early the following morning, I wondered if I would ever return. I felt very scared. There would be no comfort in store when I got home either, for I had no idea what to expect. I had never really been affected by anything terrible before. I thought of everyone forced to leave their home because of war or natural disasters. The only difference between me and them was luck.

Al-Massira Airport, Agadir, did not resemble an airport in any way that morning. It was too crowded to get any idea of what it was really like. All the Arrivals and Departures boards had been switched off. We found a piece of paper stuck to the wall. It listed a flight from our airline, but not quite at the time we had been given, and the flight number was different.

We found something resembling the start of a queue, containing other English speakers. There was no information being disseminated, but, from time to time, rumours spread through the mob like currents in a river. Occasionally, everyone would surge forward, and we would end up in a slightly different position. We were getting closer to the check-in area, so I took this as progress of a sort. It was uncertain how much our flight booking really meant. Finally, and I don't actually remember how, we ended up at the desk, and were given boarding passes. We got through Security.

The Departure Lounge was surreal. Despite everything, it held vestiges of normality. People were drinking coffee and eating overpriced baguettes, whilst others shopped for Duty Free. I was worrying, because it had never really been established whether the flight that we thought we were booked on even existed. I told myself that we all had boarding passes and so it did not really matter. But I felt that the normal rules were being eroded around me, and so, similarly, boarding passes might mean nothing.

This fear intensified when the flight was called, and we were queueing to board. People were being turned away from the gate. When it was my turn, I was shaking as they looked at my passport and boarding pass.

Finally, I got onto the plane. I still remember the smell, that particular plane smell, as I walked through the door. And the sounds: little details that I had never noticed before. As I went to take my seat, a member of the cabin crew helped me with my bag.

She smiled, and said, 'Let me. We'll look after you from now on.'

Or maybe she didn't. To be honest, I can't really remember what she said, but I do remember that the words 'look after' were in it. I gave her my bag and burst into tears. It was the first time I had let myself cry since the whole thing began.

At the end of the flight, the same flight attendant gave a little speech. I can't remember it precisely, but it went a bit like this: 'Budget airlines have a reputation for being late, but we always get you there in the end. It has been an absolute pleasure, and we are really proud to have brought you all home safely today, and I would like to thank you for your patience and positivity.'

I started crying again.

We landed in Gatwick, and said our farewells at the luggage carousel. It was an oddly anti-climactic ending to what we had been through. I got the Gatwick Express and then the tube. I wasn't sure if I was allowed to, but I didn't know the rules of the world, or the rules of London, anymore, and how else was I supposed to get home?

The next day, Friday, 20th March, was a strange one. I was not due back to work until Monday. I felt jittery and spent most of the day lying on my sofa. I kept on telling myself that I would get up and go out — but out to do what? I just couldn't seem to summon up the energy or the inclination. I found myself thinking about the flight attendant on the plane, and the effect her few, kind words had had on me. I knew how important positive, compassionate communication was. But previously I had known it from an intellectual place; now, I had experienced it from an emotional one.

## March 2020: Heading Somewhere Different

I went back to work on Monday, 23 March, the day the country was put into lockdown. In those first weeks of the pandemic, the department felt eerie and strange. It was as if it was holding its breath and waiting for something to happen.

During 'ten at ten' teaching, we focused on education around COVID. As the importance of looking after staff was being highlighted, it was decided that I should also do a wellness session on some of the mornings.

I had just read an article from the British Society of Psychologists about how to look after your team during a pandemic. They suggested that it was important that you created spaces where staff felt safe to talk about their feelings. I started the sessions, as always, with a check-in, and asked everyone to give me a number out of ten to express how they felt.

There was, paradoxical as it sounds, an odd familiarity in going round the room doing this on that day. I had done it so many times before and heard a range of emotions, both positive and negative. Now, instead of the negative emotions being tiredness and stress about having no beds, they were focused on fear about what was going to happen. But something about the familiarity of saying it out loud seemed to help contain it. As always, there was reassurance in realising that everyone felt the same way.

I had thought long and hard about what I could do next. Playing games was impossible, because of social distancing. I decided to get everyone to draw how they felt. When I handed out pens and paper, I sensed that some people felt much the same way as I had done in Morocco, when I had been told that we were still going to write each day; they felt I was asking them to do something trivial, when they should really be worrying about something big. But I had learned from experience that if you waited a few minutes, everyone would start paying attention to what they were doing.

As people concentrated, the energy became calmer. Drawing was a way of expressing things which some people found hard to articulate. Drawing together created a world in which everyone could share their experiences, without having to say too much.

I wanted to keep the drawings. I felt that they were a unique record of our experience during that time. I came up with the idea of having them made into a short film and we had a graphic designer animate them. Watching it still brings back so many memories for me. I am reminded of sitting in that room during the first wave of the pandemic, with everyone talking about how they were feeling: people discussed their fears and anxieties, and the strangeness of the time in which we were living.

Despite all the fear, there was, at times, something hopeful during that first wave. People talked about the simple pleasures they took from being outside, reconnecting with nature. A quietness had settled over London, and it brought with it an eerie beauty. The phrase the 'new normal' was used a lot. We entertained the idea that, someday, we would have a normality back again, but it would be different from the normality we had known before. We sensed that we were leaving something familiar behind, and heading for somewhere different.

## November 2022: You Can't Escape Your Problems

Two and a half years after we fled Morocco, I was off to Essaouira again for another creative writing retreat. This return trip was, in some ways, emotional for both Claire and me. I joked that it was the kind of thing that they could make a Radio 4 documentary about. However, as the time drew near, I realised that it posed exactly the same problem for me as talking at the conference had; the problem my whole life now posed: my ridiculous, pregnant shape and the danger that I might be asked about it.

Back in the summer, on one of the many occasions that I had ramped up my diet, looking nice for Essaouira had been one of the goals. It had been sufficiently far away at that time to seem achievable. Now, standing here in my flat with my suitcase waiting to be packed, I had to concede that it was yet another goal that I had failed miserably to achieve.

I hadn't been able to bear thinking about it. I just didn't have the space in my head, but the time had come, and there was no escaping from it. I felt desperately sad that I was in this position. And angry. I felt myself being dragged to the edge of the place of shame and fear. I did not have time for this. Somehow, I had to find enough clothes to wear for a week's holiday. I needed to focus.

I had checked the temperature for Morocco, and it was to be warm enough to require summer clothes. I got out several pairs of light cotton trousers that I had had made for me in India, back in a time where I believed that I had needed to lose weight, but had no idea what lay ahead for me. For a moment, I envied my old self.

To my astonishment, they fit. My belly was still huge — it dominated everything — but I must have lost some weight around my hips and my bottom. Maybe my diet was working. I just needed to be patient. I had lost weight from my arms and shoulders after all, and now it seemed to be working across my hips and bottom. Surely my belly would be next?

I felt a burst of happiness, or, at least, relief. Then the little voice in my head whispered, 'You still look pregnant.'

My reaction was a combination of sadness, anger and despair. I was so tired of my size and shape. I could think of nothing else. It was so huge inside my head and I was so huge in my body. Maybe I just had to accept that this was how I was going to look forever.

I no longer cared that I had put on weight; I just wanted not to look pregnant. And I just wanted to go away on holiday and not have to think about it. I had been looking forward to this for ages and now, like everything else, it was going to be affected by my shape. I just could not escape from it.

The day we left did not start well. I tried to get a taxi, but it took ages to find one. In the past, I would have just walked to the Underground and got the tube. But I couldn't face lugging my suitcase there. The truth was, I didn't feel physically able to carry it up and down the stairs.

Finally, I got a taxi, but it seemed to take ages to get to the station. My panic intensified. What if I missed the train, and then the plane?

By the time I got to Departures, I was a bag of nerves. The airport was uncomfortably hot. In my flat, I had convinced myself that I had disguised my shape well. I had found a very large, baggy top. Now, I felt that I simply looked like a pregnant person wearing a large, baggy top. I was nervous that some of the other women on the trip were going to ask me if I was pregnant. No-one did, but I couldn't help imagining that they were wondering. I was also anxious about getting on the plane. On my flight from Belfast, they had asked if I was pregnant. I thought this was because I was in one of the emergency exit seats, with extra leg room, so when I reserved my seat for this flight, I had made sure that I was nowhere near an emergency exit.

Other than being very uncomfortable, the flight was uneventful. However, on arrival, the airport was hot, and the queue for passport control was long. I was feeling very anxious. Even though I hadn't missed the plane, it was as if I hadn't been able to clear the anxiety that I would. Along with that, and feeling very exposed and on high alert that I might be accused of being pregnant, I was also anxious about a rather retro issue: COVID.

I had largely forgotten about COVID and so, it seemed, had the couple of countries I had travelled to in the last year. I had just assumed that Morocco had, too. However, something that was said on the plane made me think that they had not, so I was also fretting that I should have done something like take a test and have the results. When we arrived, we were given a form to complete, which asked about COVID status, contacts, and vaccination. That was all. But it whipped up my anxiety even more.

At that stage, my brain wasn't interested in the provenance or validity of what was making me anxious. It just threw everything into the big pot that was brewing in my head. Then the inevitable happened: an official directed me to a fast-track queue. I tried to shake my head, discreetly, but this just made him talk louder.

'Pregnant ladies can go through,' he kept repeating.

He didn't seem to understand when I tried to demur. I had to repeat 'Not pregnant, just fat,' several times. Finally, he went away, still bemused.

Part of me wished that I had just gone through the fast-track queue. That, though, was still the line I did not want to cross: pretending that I actually was pregnant. But I was so humiliated. One of the other women had witnessed the exchange. I tried to make a joke about it, but failed.

I just wanted to get away, but the queue was moving so slowly that it hardly seemed to be moving at all. And the room we were in was so oppressively hot. How much more of this could I take? How many more times would I be asked if I were pregnant? Would I just have to become a total recluse? Maybe I should see someone about this? Beg them to help me. Tell them I was suicidal with all these comments. It was a flippant thought, but as soon as I thought it, I realised how much I couldn't stand my situation. I couldn't live the rest of my life like this. Maybe I *would* go and see someone.

I felt myself totter at the edge of something and, from nowhere, all my fears rose up. I just felt terrified. I really needed to get away — from that Arrivals Hall, from the heat and the queue and my shame. But the line had come to a complete standstill. I strained to see what was going on or not going on. There were so many people, and even when the line started moving again, I was nowhere near the front. My mind began to spiral wildly out of control. Perhaps we had all died in a plane crash, and we were now, in fact, in purgatory. For a moment, I was amused that the afterlife was asking about COVID. Then I started to feel like I might faint.

Back in school, I had been a fainter. Well, that's not exactly true; it's a bit more complex than that. I first fainted at primary school, at the end of assembly. It was a Protestant primary school in Northern Ireland in the seventies, so we sang the National Anthem. I had felt strange, but I thought that I should wait until the end of *God Save the Queen* before I told a teacher. On and on it went, and I felt stranger and stranger. Then everything changed and I realised that, somehow, I was lying on the floor, and everyone was looking down at me.

I was told that I had fainted. I found this quite novel. I had, of course, seen people faint on TV but never in real life. It made me feel special. My parents were called and came to take me home.

The second time I fainted was at grammar school and, yet again, it was in assembly. I can't remember if we sang the National Anthem there or not. I began to feel strange, and then I thought, 'This is the feeling I got when I fainted as a child.' Then I was on the floor, and everyone was looking down at me. Once again, my parents were called. I was sent home from school and immediately sent to bed. It is unclear whether I was ill or just overtired. I had been staying up very late, studying for exams.

Then, not long after that, a strange thing happened in assembly. I felt perfectly well but suddenly, for no reason, I began to think about fainting. It was an idle thought but then it became more panicky. I remembered what it felt like to faint. I remembered it so vividly that it became hard for me to know whether I was really going to faint or was just imagining it. I didn't want to cause a fuss if it was all in my imagination. I wasn't sure how to judge it. I began to fidget. I must have been spotted by one of the teachers, because I was beckoned out of the room. The minute I sat down, I felt more normal. I must have imagined it all. I felt dreadful that I had caused a scene.

After that, I became scared of going into assembly. I wasn't sure how to tell the difference between a real feeling and an imagined one. At what point should I call for help? Had I really been about to faint, or had I just imagined it? Or, even more confusing, had I somehow made what was occurring in my imagination real?

In the queue for passport control in Essaouira, I began to fidget, moving around to get the blood flowing, sipping from my bottle of now tepid water, fanning myself with my passport. But none of it worked. My peripheries were tingling; I was sweating profusely and felt that distinctive combination of cold and clammy. Just like at school, I didn't know at what point I should call it. I really didn't want to cause a fuss, particularly if it was all in my imagination. I didn't want to draw attention to myself. Especially looking the way that I did. If I fainted, everyone would assume that I was pregnant.

In the end, I had to concede defeat. I lay down on the ground. The relief was immeasurable. I'm not sure if I did black out for a few minutes or not. But I closed my eyes and let the feeling pass.

Obviously, there was a huge fuss. Someone appeared from the crowd who was a doctor. I told him that I was fine, and I was a doctor too. He told me I was a patient now. I tried to roll over towards my front. I really didn't want him to see my belly and start asking questions. Mercifully, he didn't. When I was well enough, I was ushered through the fast door: the one that they had tried to send me through at the beginning. I was deeply embarrassed and sorry for having caused a whole lot of bother.

On the transfer into Essaouira, I should have felt excited. But I just felt very sad. I had absolutely no idea how I was going to get through the week.

## November 2022: Another Lockdown

That night, in bed, I realised that I was going to have to manage my holiday pretty much the same way that I managed my life in London. Basically, I couldn't go out much; I just couldn't risk it. I had an image of wandering round the souk and everyone asking me about my imminent baby; worse, wandering round the souk, with other people in the group witnessing me, on multiple occasions, having to explain that I wasn't pregnant. I imagined them getting sucked into the embarrassment of it all, dreading it as much as I did. Thinking about that filled me with horror.

So, I just stayed in the hotel. It was the first holiday in my life that I didn't do any shopping. It was pretty easy. We all wrote together in the mornings and then the afternoons were free. Some people went off in small groups for lunch, but there were always two or three who did their own thing. I said that I wanted to do some writing. It was a creative writing retreat after all, and people would do that. Also, I was working on a novel, so it made perfect sense. I skipped lunch as I felt that even going out to get something to eat was too risky. I told myself that it was good for my diet.

In the evening, I generally joined the others for dinner, but on a few nights a couple of people decided to stay back in the hotel and so, on those occasions, I stayed with them. That turned to be an unexpected highlight; we had some really good conversations.

I tried to be positive. The hotel itself was very beautiful: two old riads, joined together. It was like its own little world, walled off from the outside. Now, it became my little world also. I told myself that I had come to write, and this was a great opportunity to finish my novel. But as I listened to the sound of the others leaving for lunch, I felt very sad as I heard their laughter disappear. It was as if all the joy was seeping from my life. My shape was exiling me from it. It was forcing me into the life of a recluse. I felt odd and not myself.

I'm an extrovert and have always loved being part of a group, but now I was excluding myself from one. It was as if I existed only on the periphery. It was an unpleasant place for someone of my temperament to be. It affected my confidence too. My shape had eroded everything that was important to me in life. It had taken away my Zumba classes, going out and socialising, and now it was robbing me of my ability to enjoy holidays. I had always loved going on holiday — it was my ultimate treat — and now I feared that I might never feel comfortable doing it again.

I had last been in Essaouira when it began to lock down. It hit me, with a bitter irony, that I had had more freedom then than I had now. My stupid shape and all the comments that went with it were keeping me more of a prisoner than a global pandemic had: I was enduring my own private lockdown. The only thing that I had left was writing. Obviously, writing is important to me: that was why I was on a creative writing retreat. I had written every day since the start of the pandemic. But it felt to me, on that trip, that something magical happened with my writing. Perhaps it was having so much time and so few distractions. Perhaps it was because so much was simmering away inside me, so much about what had been happening to me and my body, all mixed up with what had been happening at work, and my writing was the only way out. It was like the valve on a pressure cooker.

Perhaps it was because I hated my self-imposed isolation so much that I loved writing with the group in the morning. I would soak up all their energy and creativity like cracked, hard earth soaks up the rain. Then I would take it all back to my room and create my own world, inside which I could exist, as I was now too scared to be part of the world outside.

## November 2022: What Is a Little Knowledge?

While we were away, one of the other writers did ask me if I was pregnant.

'No,' I sighed, wearily. 'It's just the menopause.'

She agreed that the menopause was indeed a cruel thing. 'But maybe you should get it checked out,' she added. 'It's probably nothing, but it might be a good idea.'

There it was again: someone telling me to get it checked out. I felt that icy drip, drip of fear.

I hadn't really looked at myself since Belfast. Even in my hotel in Berlin, I had managed to avoid my appearance most of the time. In my head, I had almost separated myself from my body; I had tried to disown it mentally. We might have to co-exist, but I tried to have nothing else to do with it.

But here, trapped in a hotel room with a full mirror, it was impossible to ignore my body. My reflection seemed to have changed again, but I wasn't quite sure how. I looked comically grotesque, not like a real person at all. Unclothed, there was definitely something odd about my appearance. I reminded myself of someone from a medical textbook. The whiteness of my room gave a cold, clinical background to my reflection. Something about the sterility of it made it all more chilling. I looked like I should have pixelated features or blacked-out eyes.

What were the causes of abdominal distension again? Medicine is all lists: long lists of things we have to remember and are then examined on. There was certainly a list for abdominal distension. For a moment, I got it confused with the causes of cholecystitis, as they both contain a lot of things which begin with F, and fat is in each of them. Then I remembered the distension list: fat, fluid, foetus, flatus, fibroid.

Maybe I had a fibroid, I thought. I had heard of women having fibroids so big that they looked pregnant. But I had never had any other symptoms of fibroids. And fibroids were supposed to get smaller after the menopause. Maybe some didn't, but I couldn't see that a menopausal woman would suddenly develop a fibroid so huge that it was making her look like this.

Fluid was another cause. The medical term for this is ascites and there was, indeed, something about my appearance that reminded me of a patient with ascites. But the commonest cause of ascites is liver failure and, surely, if I had liver failure I would be jaundiced? I certainly wasn't yellow. This was ridiculous. I didn't have liver failure and I didn't have jaundice. I lay down and felt my stomach. What are you doing? I asked myself; you are being ridiculous. My stomach didn't feel like any ascites I had felt before. As a junior doctor, I had drained ascites from patients. Nowadays, we use ultrasound, but back then we just had to palpate the abdomen. You could feel the fluid moving. I remembered one patient whose ascites we drained every other day for a month. She had liver failure and was profoundly jaundiced. For a moment, I wondered what had happened to her. She had probably died, I thought, and felt a little shiver.

I felt my abdomen. It didn't feel like ascites. For a start, it was rock hard. I had noticed this a while back. I put it down to gaining visceral fat rather than subcutaneous fat. Another menopause thing. No, I wouldn't like to stick a needle in that. For good measure, I tested to see if I had a fluid thrill. This is one of the tests for ascites: you flick the abdomen on one side and if there is fluid there, it should travel like a wave over to the other side. There was no fluid thrill in my hard abdomen.

But I wasn't fully reassured. My appearance unsettled me as much as it disgusted me. Another afternoon, I googled causes of abdominal distension, just to make sure I hadn't forgotten anything. Doctors use Dr Google too. There was my list, with the addition of a sixth F — filthy great tumour or, some had it, fucking great tumour. Ah, that old medical student humour, always finding ways of sneaking a profanity into a list or mnemonic.

Did I have a filthy great tumour? Is that what was causing my filthy great abdomen? I read on. As I suspected, the tumour caused the distension not by itself, but by producing fluid: ascites. The commonest causes were ovarian tumour and a tumour of the gastro-intestinal tract. Development of ascites was a poor prognostic indicator. According to Dr Google, survival rate of longer than three months was rare.

Get a grip, I told myself. Firstly, the notion that I had ascites was preposterous. Also, I had had this problem for much longer than three months. People had first commented on the fact that I looked pregnant in April, six months previously, and I had looked big before that. I remembered how long I had been so big and, ironically, it brought me some relief. The idea that I had been walking around for months, maybe even a year — going to work and doing my Zumba — with ascites and a filthy great tumour was frankly ridiculous.

I felt somewhat reassured. But still something niggled away at me, and that something was the now defunct MRCP Part 1. 'What are the causes of massive ascites?' sounded like a question from the exam. Was there another list somewhere? A list that I had never committed properly to memory...

Of course, the question wouldn't have been put in quite such simple terms. Why only test people on rare medical conditions that they had never heard of when you could catch them out on semantics too? It would have been worded 'Massive ascites is most commonly caused by...' so that if you did happen to have memorised a list of causes, you would wonder if they were common causes or just causes. Or they might phrase it as 'Rare causes of massive ascites include...' with a list of lots of obscure conditions like tropical sprue that no-one had ever heard of, let alone seen.

I went to google it. Stop it, I told myself. You are on holiday; stop trying to google questions from an extinct exam to try and diagnose yourself. Go and see your GP when you get back. You are just fat, but maybe they will be able to help with that. I took one last look at my huge belly in the mirror.

## November 2022: Rome Didn't Fall in a Day

When I got back from Morocco, I felt sad. I had looked forward to it for so long and I was disappointed that things had ended up the way that they had. Once I was home, I felt reluctant to see my GP. I had just put on weight; I was being overdramatic. I decided that I would try harder with my diet.

'How, how, how?' said the little voice in my head.

'You can always try harder,' I replied. 'There is always room for improvement, isn't there?'

'Insanity is trying the same thing and expecting a different result, if we want to trade sayings,' muttered the little voice.

Anyway, I *was* losing weight, I told myself, just not from where I needed to lose it. It seemed to be coming off everywhere but my belly. Surely it was only a matter of time, if I was really, really strict.

'Perhaps the GP could help with weight loss?' suggested the little voice.

In the end, I made a deal with myself: I would try my super-strict diet until Christmas and if that didn't work, then I would concede defeat and see my GP in the new year.

November became December. Work was truly, truly horrendous. It had been horrendous for some time. But, every now and then, it would surprise me by becoming even more horrendous. The press pointed out that every winter the NHS said that it was on the verge of collapse, and it always survived. This felt different, though.

I had always thought of the collapse of the NHS as threatening some point in the future. But now I realised that this was it: the NHS was collapsing around us. It suddenly hit me: just as Rome hadn't fallen in a day, neither would the NHS.

There wasn't a specific day in history, taught to successive generations, when the Roman Empire officially ended. There wasn't a date when they handed over control to the Saxons, Goths and Vandals. Similarly, there would be no final day for the NHS. No date where we would announce a leaving party or a closing down sale. It would just disintegrate. And that is what was happening now.

Out there on the edges, in the Emergency Department, we were already trying to dodge the debris as it crashed down around us. Every single day was nightmarish. The overcrowding was appalling; there was no space anywhere. When I doom-scrolled on Twitter, I could see that throughout the whole country, the NHS was in the same old leaky boat. We were all trying to go about our day-to-day business as it sank.

Some hospitals adapted their corridors to make it easier to care for patients in them. Other people responded that this was just normalising the situation. Every hospital had ambulances stacked outside. I read of some places where the wait even to get into hospital was twelve hours. It seemed a luxury to be able to see a patient in a cubicle. With the darkest and bitterest of humour, we joked that we didn't just have corridor medicine, we also had carpark medicine. In fact, one of the suggestions to the problem in some places was to erect tents in the carpark, in which to see people.

I hated having to attend to patients inside ambulances. Firstly, my size and shape made climbing in and out of them very difficult. Once inside, I felt uncomfortable and was even more aware of my hugeness in the confined space. Every bit of me seemed to ache in the freezing cold. Also, it was hard to switch to working in such an unfamiliar environment. Safety depends on familiarity, and the difference in environment added yet another level of risk. The whole situation seemed barbaric.

One day, I saw a lady who was in her eighties. The wait to unload ambulances was several hours. It was icy outside, and I offered to go and see if I could find her a blanket in the department.

'Oh no, dear, don't you worry about that. I can imagine you must be very busy. These boys are looking after me very well.' She nodded towards the two paramedics.

'Can I just say how sorry I am,' I said, 'that we are having to treat you in this way? It's probably of no comfort to you at all, but let me reassure you that none of us want to be practising medicine like this.'

The paramedics nodded in agreement.

'In fact, I am appalled and deeply ashamed that I am having to do this,' I added. I felt my eyes and nose tingle in that way that they do when you are about to cry.

The patient reached out and took my hand. 'Don't you worry, love,' she said. 'You have absolutely nothing to apologise for.'

She gave my hand a little squeeze and I braced myself for some sort of comment of how getting upset wasn't good for me or the baby.

'We just all have to make sure that we vote the fuckers out at the next election,' she said.

## December 2022: Schrödinger's Dieter

If all that wasn't bad enough, the next thing we got hit with was Group A streptococcus, a bacterial infection that causes a number of conditions, including scarlet fever in children. It can, on occasions, lead to serious infections and even result in death.

Often it will start with a sore throat, high temperature and just feeling miserable. Unfortunately, so do many other harmless viral infections common in winter. The Group A strep outbreak had tragically already resulted in child fatalities. This, understandably, resulted in many parents bringing sick children to us. Paediatric attendances almost quadrupled at the worst point that December. You can imagine adding up to four times the normal number of children and their parents into an already overcrowded department. It was relentless. It was already relentless, of course. This just made it more so.

Waiting times got even longer and tempers got even more frayed. As always, some of this erupted into violence, most of which was directed at the staff. The nightshifts were exceptionally bad. People were verbally abused on a regular basis. It's easy to dismiss verbal abuse as just people shouting at you. But it's much worse than that. If you get called 'stupid bitch' or 'fat cunt' on a regular basis, it does more than momentarily hurt your feelings.

Due to my size, I felt particularly unwilling to put myself in the firing line. The irony is that I was probably protected by the fact that most people assumed that I was pregnant. That only protected me from being called fat, though: not from any of the other abuse. I have seen heavily pregnant nurses abused on numerous occasions, up to the point where people have threatened to punch them in the stomach and hope that it kills the baby.

Verbal abuse on top of everything else that you are trying to deal with can push you over the edge. And when it happens, there is usually no time to deal with it; you are just required to go on and see the next patient.

It doesn't stop with verbal abuse, though. Hate crime is rife in emergency departments. Staff are regularly racially or homophobically abused. Racial abuse has been shown to have long-term adverse health effects, increasing the risk of illness and premature death.

Then it moves into physical assault. Staff report being spat at, having things thrown at them and threatened with worse.

We tried to support people as best we could, but I feared that it just wasn't enough. We really needed to be doing more to stop it happening in the first place, but what *could* we do? Our security team was great and really protected us. We also encouraged people to report any crime — hate crime, threatening behaviour or physical assaults — to the police, and we spoke regularly to our liaison officers at the staff safety meetings. But none of that helped the situation on any given night.

Predictably, sickness rates soared, and lack of staffing worsened. Every hospital in the country was in the same boat, which was leaking even more dramatically now.

It seemed to me that between work and my attempts to diet and lose my huge belly, life was just a series of vicious circles, spinning faster and faster and reducing my room for manoeuvre. My body and I seemed to be two different entities, forced together. Every morning I would look at the dome of my belly under the covers and wonder why I was now this person.

I was sticking to my super diet. It was surprisingly easy. For once, the promise that, after a few days, I wouldn't feel hungry seemed to hold up. I felt surprisingly full when I ate and if I did feel hungry in the afternoons, a couple of dates satisfied me. But as to whether it was working, it was very hard to say.

I was certainly losing weight; I could easily feel my ribs but, below them, my belly remained enormous. Again, some days, I thought that it looked like it was getting bigger, but I surmised that this was some kind of optical illusion as I was getting smaller everywhere else. I was like Schrödinger's dieter, simultaneously getting bigger and smaller at the same time. I was permanently exhausted. When I got up in the mornings, the only thing that kept me going was looking forward to going to bed again that night. I had always been the sort of person who could easily sit up until midnight, but now I started going to bed earlier and earlier. The earliest was seven thirty. I told myself that I would watch TV, but I fell asleep immediately. But I was no different from anyone else at work. We were all exhausted.

Work was even more of a struggle. Part of it was the sheer exhaustion. But there was more to it than that. I began to understand the physicality of pregnancy. My huge belly was affecting my posture and my movement. I had adopted a much more broad-based gait to balance things out. I now waddled as my huge abdomen threw itself forward and bent my back. It felt as if my stomach was leading and the rest of me following behind.

Getting up and down was a challenge too. I could no longer do it in one movement. I had to push myself up, or sometimes change position to be able to stand. Even rolling over in bed was difficult.

My shape and size made it hard for me to manoeuvre myself round the little space we had in the department. I had to squash myself into all the nooks and crannies where we were now seeing patients. If I was trying to manage someone in the corridor, people would invariably bump into me and my hard belly would bang uncomfortably against the side of the trolley. As soon as I walked into a cubicle, I was aware of a patient staring at my swollen stomach. If there were relatives present, they immediately jumped up to give me a seat.

I was permanently hyper-conscious of my size and shape. My hand frequently knocked against my belly, and it felt rock hard. It wasn't painful, but it was uncomfortable being that size. Walking any distance was a challenge, and climbing the steps to my flat overwhelmed me on occasions.

Often, I had to lie down to recover and I struggled to get up again. But I forced myself to walk home from work and often to work as well. I feared that if I got out of the habit, then that would be it: I would be doing no exercise at all.

The weekend that I worked in December was nightmarish. We were exceptionally busy and overcrowded and very short-staffed. I don't know how I managed to keep going. At one point, a patient collapsed in the corridor, and I really struggled to kneel down to see to them. I can only describe the efforts of the whole team as heroic.

When I got home that Sunday night, I was too tired to do anything, including eat. I wasn't hungry anyway. As I sat there, scrolling through Twitter, I came across a tweet. It was by a medical journalist who had been in the department that day. He praised the staff for the way they had carried on delivering excellent care in very difficult circumstances. When I saw it, I immediately emailed it to the team, and then cried. I must have cried for about an hour; I was unable to stop.

Maybe I was burnt-out and needed time off work. But even the thought of trying to organise that was too much. I felt as if everything was closing in around me. It was like being in one of those horror films where the doors and the ceiling start moving, and the room shrinks. There was no space; I was being squashed in everywhere.

Everything was getting smaller, except for my belly which was getting larger. I was like Alice in Wonderland when she starts growing and fills up the room. I felt as if I were being forced down a long, dark tunnel and it was getting narrower and narrower.

One night, as I was getting into bed, I caught a glimpse of my shadow flitting against the wall. It looked bizarre; a great big ball balanced on spindly limbs. It was grotesque; it didn't even look quite human. It was monstrous, but at the same time there was something almost comical about it, like a creature from a shadow puppet theatre.

## 2020/2021: Out of the Shadows

An unexpected consequence of COVID was that *everyone* began talking about staff wellness, and, for once, resources were being directed towards it. Many places gave a huge boost to the 'basics': those facilities that are fundamental in any good workplace but are frequently woefully inadequate in the NHS. They can be as simple as lockers, shower facilities and bike racks, but they just smooth out the experience of being at work.

One thing which has long been a bugbear of mine is the almost universal lack of provision of twenty-four-hour access to food for staff, even though staff provide a twenty-four-hour service. Many hospital canteens close around 5pm. I once mentioned this to someone senior in the NHS, whose response was 'Surely they can just bring in their own food?' This lack of interest in making people's lives easier infuriated me. It is hard to organise bringing food to work, particularly on nightshifts, and particularly if you're also trying to organise your children, as many people are.

It also overlooked the fact that many departments no longer had access to microwaves or fridges. Appropriate rest areas for staff had been another casualty of cutbacks over the years. I think this stands as a good visual indicator of how organisations view their staff.

The lack of food angered me for other, deeper reasons too. There is such a fundamental link between food and love, between food and caring, between food and the desire to nourish. An organisation that cares about its staff should care about feeding them.

As it happened, our solution to the problem of twenty-four-hour food provision came during the pandemic. Alick Varma lived locally to the hospital and, like many people, wanted to do his bit to support the NHS. He asked local restaurants if they would like to prepare meals that he would deliver to hospitals in the area. The restaurants were closed, and although many of their staff were on furlough, they too wanted to do their bit. He told me that everyone was immensely proud to support the NHS.

Alick Varma noticed how positively the food was received. So, when the charity funding was coming to an end, he sent out a questionnaire asking if staff would be willing to pay for the food. Over 90% of people responded with a yes. From that, he devised his *Meals for the NHS* smart fridges.

The first fridge was such a success that the hospital bought more. I am proud that I got the second one into the Emergency Department tearoom. Of all my interventions for staff wellbeing, this might be the most successful.

Not long after the fridge had been installed, one of our nurses told me that, when she was doing long days, she sometimes bought food from the fridge at the end of her shift and took it home for the family meal. Her children all loved it. She asked if I minded. Not only did I not mind, I was delighted. After working an intense twelve-hour shift, going home and caring for your family is, no doubt, exhausting. I was pleased that the fridge was not just making people's lives easier inside work, but also outside work.

Another pandemic initiative was Project Wingman, begun by Dave Fielding and Emma Henderson, both of whom were airline workers. They came up with the idea of setting up 'first class' lounges in hospitals. Staffed by volunteers furloughed from the airline industry, they were somewhere for NHS staff to relax and decompress. This was particularly important where staff no longer had a proper rest area. The Project Wingman team understood that people who care need to be cared for. I felt myself frequently drawn there, particularly in the first terrifying weeks of the pandemic.

It's easy now to forget how scared we all were. But we were. At work, we had no idea what was going to happen to us, or if we would be able to cope. Outside work was frightening, too. Everything felt strange: queuing outside supermarkets, having to stay in most of the time, taking just one walk a day, through deserted streets. And we were scared that we would die, or end up in Intensive Care, like the people we saw, the same age as us and younger.

One of my nursing colleagues was impressed by the communication skills of the airline staff. There is an established correlation between pilots and clinicians, who are responsible for client and patient safety. However, to my knowledge, no-one had previously conceived of learning from the cabin crew. It struck us that we had a lot in common and that we could learn from each other. Airline passengers had similarities with Emergency Department patients: both groups were often anxious and/or scared.

Airlines understood the importance of communicating well from the beginning. They knew that if they didn't, passengers were more likely to become angry, aggressive, or even violent, mid-air.

Some of the volunteers from Project Wingman formed a company called WingFactors, to deliver courses based around combined expertise from aviation and medicine. I worked with Wayne McCormack, a cabin crew manager and educator, and Alex Jolly and Dave Fielding, the other founders of WingFactors, to design a course around positive communication. We devised a series of modules relevant to both Emergency Department staff and NHS staff in other specialties. Content included how to create a good first impression and how to manage expectations. My role was to act as a bridge between the world of medicine and the world of aviation.

We ran our very first course on 19th March, 2021, which, by coincidence, was the first anniversary of my flight back from Morocco. We continued to develop and run the course during 2022.

Within the NHS, people felt guarded optimism. We had learned lessons from the pandemic and understood more clearly what we were capable of. There was a feeling that we could not, and should not, go backwards. This was our opportunity to change things for the better, and it was particularly true regarding staff wellness, which was now something that everyone was talking about. Surely, now it had been brought out of the shadows, there was no way that it could be pushed back into them again?

## December 2022: A New Place

I avoided all social occasions that Christmas. Thankfully, I was scheduled to work on the night of the Christmas party, so that made things easier. I had nothing to wear and no desire to be seen in public either.

I was back to trying to avoid my own body. A couple of times when I woke, I had the oddest sensation in my upper abdomen, just below my ribs. It was like a stretching feeling. The first time, I was worried that I had grown even larger overnight. I forced myself to look in the mirror. My reflection was disconcerting. Previously, it had just been horrible to look at. Now, it was *difficult* to look at.

A few people commented that I appeared to have lost weight. But I took no satisfaction. Something in their tone was not quite normal. Nothing about the way they said it sounded complimentary. One or two people followed it up by asking if I was alright. I said I was fine, apart from work. Then I would give a little laugh, to make a joke about it.

One morning, walking to work, three teenagers came towards me.

'Look at that woman,' I heard one of them say, as if she was drawing attention to something odd. 'Is she pregnant?' She sounded uncertain.

As they got near, they called out to me, 'Are you pregnant?'

I nodded wearily.

'Congratulations,' they all shouted, as they went past.

I didn't care that I was pretending. It didn't seem quite so clear cut anymore. Being pregnant seemed to be the lesser of two evils. I no longer looked like any version of normal; I was starting to look freaky.

## December 2022: Defeated

I no longer hated Christmas, as I had done in the first years after my father's death, but I didn't particularly like it either. I had taken it off work when my nephew was small, but for the last ten years I had chosen to work. Traditionally, Christmas Day was quiet, but on the previous two years it had been a nightmare, due to COVID, overcrowding and understaffing.

Staffing was a problem, as few people wanted to work during that time. This had been an issue for the past decade, but we had coped. Now, when it was so busy, we couldn't manage with that level of understaffing. After Christmas 2021, I had joked that I was done; I couldn't go through another one. Like many jokes that I make, the more I said it, the more I realised that there was some truth in it. So, in 2022, I requested leave.

I normally made an effort to do festive things for the team, but I couldn't be bothered. I didn't try and make sure someone put up decorations; I didn't arrange a secret Santa; I didn't go to the Christmas party. I just counted down the days until I could go home.

It felt as if everything had closed in around me: my life was just one long, dark tunnel, and I was crawling along on my hands and knees. I was bitterly aware that my extreme diet hadn't worked, and Christmas had been my deadline. My body had defeated me.

Just before I went home, both my shower and my washing machine broke. I didn't have the energy, either mental or physical, to sort them out. My entire flat was a mess, but I was too tired to do anything about it. My whole life was broken, and I didn't know how to fix it.

I felt an immense relief when I arrived home. I was really happy to be back with my family. Perhaps the last two years of COVID had changed things in some way. I was so grateful to be where I was and not at work trying to deal with all the awfulness.

Christmas Day was great. I joked that my mother, sister, nephew and I managed to make the Christmas dinner together and didn't want to kill each other. We didn't fight at all. I was anxious about having to eat so much food — I was used to not eating very much — but I managed a medium-sized plate. Afterwards, I was very aware of the hardness I felt in my belly.

Often, when I am at home in the winter, I find myself going a bit stir-crazy. The winter weather on the North Coast is not particularly conducive to making you want to leave the house. That Christmas, I was grateful for it. I had no desire to do anything, and the rain and wind gave me an excuse not to. I was happy to sleep late in the morning and go out for a drive in the afternoon. Occasionally, I saw my mother looking at me strangely.

I must be one of the few people in the country who likes New Year's Eve. I always go out with my friend, Alison. We have been close friends since school. This year, though, I said that I couldn't go out as I was exhausted. Also, I had to fly back to London on 1st January, and I didn't think I could manage to do that after being out the night before. This was partly true. I also didn't have anything to wear, naturally, and I did not want anyone to see me looking the way that I did.

I was sad to cancel. New Year has always been important to me since my father died. Firstly, it marks the end of the festive period, which I found a cause for celebration. Secondly, it has always represented something to do with new beginnings. I find New Year a hopeful occasion.

I remembered the previous New Year and all my good intentions, and how I had decided to lose weight. I felt very depressed about how I looked now. I nearly changed my mind a couple of times, but I just couldn't go through with it. It was yet another thing that my shape had taken from me.

## December 2022: Nowhere to Hide

As we couldn't go out on New Year's Eve, Alison and I arranged to meet for dinner on 29th December. She collected me, and parked ten minutes from the restaurant, close to a headland called Ramore Head. It was a stormy night, and the wind was blowing against us. I struggled to keep up with Alison. She is tall and a fast walker. At one point, I felt so bad that I thought that I was going to have to ask her to stop. I feared that if I didn't sit down, I would collapse.

I looked over towards the outline of Ramore Head in the darkness. This was an area I had walked all my life. I had come home for a week in September 2021 and walked across it every morning. How had I become so unfit in such a short period of time? I felt so unfit now that I could not imagine getting back to anything approaching what I once was.

There must be something seriously wrong, said the voice in my head.

I made it to the restaurant and struggled into my seat. Alison asked me how I was, and I told her that I was tired, very tired. After about five minutes, I began to feel normal; that is to say: the new normal; the new shit normal. I pushed all thoughts of the old normal from my head and got on with it. I was well-practised at it.

When I got home, I could sense my mother watching me. She had been watching me since I had arrived and now she was watching me very carefully. She watched me as I delicately sat down and moved myself around to find a comfortable position. She watched me as I rubbed my upper back.

'Is your back sore?' she asked.

She had asked this several times over the previous few days. It wasn't; what was sore was my rib cage, due to the fact that my ribs were now so bony that it was uncomfortable to lie in bed.

'You've put a lot of weight on round your middle,' she continued.

No, I thought, no. I just can't face having this conversation now. This isn't the right time. But I never wanted to have this conversation, so really there was no right time. I knew that I had put on weight; what did it matter to everyone else?

'I know,' I said. 'It's my age. I've tried everything. I've really tried, really, really tried.'

'And you look terrible,' she went on. 'You are emaciated around your arms and face.'

'What? I've put on weight, *and* I'm emaciated. I have to be one or the other. Make up your mind — which one am I? I can't be both.'

But I sort of was both. It was confusing me, too. And now my confusion was out in the open; it had found its voice.

'Maybe you should see a doctor,' my mother said.

No matter what age you are, something happens when you talk to your parents. The adult-you fades away, leaving a you from a much earlier time. The layers of you that remain since childhood become exposed like something from an archaeological dig.

'Why?' I asked. 'To tell them I'm fat? I don't want to see a doctor.'

'You don't look normal,' my mother persisted.

I was furious. I knew I didn't look normal. I hadn't looked normal for some time. I had tried so hard to conceal it. Carrying around my abnormality was wearing me out. My belly was like some sort of parasite that had drained me of all my physical and mental energy. It never seemed satisfied. But it was my secret and now it was being exposed.

Anyway, why couldn't I just be left alone to look not normal? It wasn't my fault I looked this way. Adolescent-me wanted an argument. I was spoiling for the sort of fight we used to have when I wanted to wear my DM boots with a skirt.

'You look pregnant,' continued my mother. 'You move like I did when I was pregnant.'

I couldn't believe it. Was there nowhere I was safe from this?

'Maybe there's something wrong with you,' she said.

'Like what?' I replied.

The irony didn't escape me. Me, the doctor, asking my non–doctor mother to tell me what was wrong with me.

My mother thought that I might have a cyst on my ovary. She had heard of people having cysts that grew to the size of melons. She knew of someone with a cyst, and it had made them look pregnant.

I tried to explain that one of the reasons that my belly looked so big was that I was dieting very hard and had lost weight from everywhere else. That is also why I looked so emaciated. It was very confusing, but I was trying so hard to lose the weight around my belly.

'But maybe it isn't weight,' repeated my mother. 'Maybe it's something else.' She looked close to tears. The adult inside me didn't want to upset her. But the child in me said, 'Like what?' My mother didn't know, but she repeated that I looked pregnant.

'Maybe you have a cyst,' she said again.

According to her, I looked like I had something growing inside me. This made me really angry. It was such a ridiculous suggestion. And behind that there was the icy drip, drip, drip of fear.

'I'm just fat,' I told her.

I felt confused. I wasn't quite sure how the argument had got to this point. We seemed to have changed positions and I was the one now telling my mother that I was fat and not the other way around. And so, we went round and round in circles: fat, emaciated, dreadful, pregnant, doctor, cyst... round and round, never finding the point. But there was a point in there somewhere: a sharp, little point that I could feel pricking away at me.

Finally, we went to bed. We were both too exhausted to continue the conversation. I wasn't even sure what we were talking about anymore.

Was my mother saying that I was fat or not?

Was I saying that I was fat or not?

Before I went to sleep, I googled causes of abdominal distension again. There they were, all six of them; all starting with F and the last one being fucking great tumour. I re-read it. If I had abdominal distension due to a fucking great tumour, then it would be caused by ascites. And having ascites associated with a huge tumour is a very poor prognostic indicator. People are sick with it. I could not have been walking around, going to work, with ascites since April. Since before April.

I suddenly remembered wearing something that I had thought made me look pregnant the previous November. I had hated it at the time. Now the memory flooded me with relief. I couldn't have had a fucking great tumour with ascites for over a year and been as well as I was. Yes, I was tired, but every single person at work was tired.

'You don't have a fucking great tumour,' I reassured myself.

In the new, confused world in which I currently existed, I felt suddenly glad that I had simply put on a lot of weight. But I had to concede defeat on what I could do to lose it. Maybe I should see my GP, I told myself.

The next afternoon I went out with my mum and my sister. We were in a furniture shop, and I caught a glimpse of myself in a mirror. It was part of a display for a bedroom for a little girl, all sparkly pink and surrounded by lightbulbs. I looked shocking. Perhaps, after the previous evening's conversation, I had let go of something. Or maybe it was that I no longer had the energy to try and convince myself that there wasn't something strange going on with my body. I was too worn out to keep up the deception. My face was skeletal, and my shoulders had all but disappeared. My chest area was sunken. My mother was right, I did look emaciated. Except, of course, for my belly. I could feel its hardness when my hand brushed against it. It was rigid and tense, and I could feel that, even through the layers of my thick puffer coat. I could no longer hide from it. The cat was out of the bag.

## January 2023: Back in London

I went back to London and back to work. I had told my mother that I would speak to my GP, but I felt a familiar reluctance. It wasn't that I wasn't going to do it; I would do it when I got round to doing it.

That's what I snapped at my mother when she phoned two nights in a row to check 'how I was'. The phone calls brought out the inner teenager in me again, and that made me even more determined not to do it. Or maybe they didn't. Maybe they just gave me an excuse for why I wasn't doing it. The cat may have been out of the bag, but it was surprisingly easy to ignore.

On the Friday, I woke from a vivid dream. I have had vivid dreams since childhood. I believe that dreams are one of the ways that your subconscious tries to communicate with you. Your subconscious often does this in a way that is difficult to understand. But it's always trying to send you the answer to problems or point out something important that you have not noticed. I used to do a cryptic crossword every evening. If I didn't complete it, I would frequently dream of things which turned out to be the answers to the clues I hadn't got. Your subconscious often knows what your conscious mind doesn't, or what it does know but won't admit.

In the dream, I was chatting to a doctor who used to work in the department. He was telling me that he couldn't swim. This embarrassed him, and he generally kept it a secret. I had never learned to swim when I was young either. I had a frightening experience as a child and could potentially have drowned and was always anxious about it after that.

'The thing is,' I said, in my dream. 'I understand your embarrassment.

I kept the fact that I couldn't swim a secret, too. Then, one day, I realised that I was deeply ashamed about it. But I started to talk about it and then I decided to confront it and took some adult swimming classes.'

'So, you can swim now?' the doctor asked me in my dream.

'After a fashion,' I replied, 'but, actually, what I discovered was that I didn't really like swimming.'

In my dream, I laughed. 'But I did stop feeling ashamed and that was the main thing. Taking those classes was one of the best things that I ever did,' my dream-self continued. 'They freed me from my shame and my fear.'

The part about being ashamed that I couldn't swim and learning as an adult was all true. As for the conversation, that had never happened. I have absolutely no idea whether he could swim or not. He was someone that I had not thought about since he stopped working with us and why my subconscious decided to pluck him out of my memory and give him a starring role in that particular dream is anyone's guess.

I may not have known why my subconscious had done that but, I knew exactly what it was trying to tell me. And, more importantly, I knew what I had to do. It spoke to me with such clarity, I could ignore it no longer. Before any other part of me had time to talk me out of it, I called the surgery. The receptionist was so lovely, she made me cry with relief.

'Is it an emergency?' she asked.

'No. I've had the symptoms a while, but I do need to be checked out.'

She could give me an appointment in a week's time, if that suited.

That was fine. I had lived with my huge belly for so long, I could wait another week. I imagined the little voice in my head cheering.

'At last,' it was saying. 'At last. I have only been trying to get through to you for the best part of a year.'

In the week leading up to my appointment, I really began to struggle. Or perhaps it was that I began to notice how much I was struggling. Now I had decided to see a GP, it felt like I didn't have to work so hard to convince myself that there was nothing wrong with me.

I struggled to get out of bed in the morning. And once I was at work,

I struggled to do anything. When I sat down, I found it very hard to get up again. I spent as much of my clinical shift as I could sitting on a chair and discussing patients with the juniors.

Some people may argue that that week I was at my best as a consultant. I spent lots of time teaching rather than rushing around. At least when I tried to teach people, they appreciated what I was doing. In an odd sort of way, I actually began to have moments when I started to enjoy the job again. I saw snatches of why I had fallen in love with it in the first place.

One morning, one of the juniors came to me with a query about a patient with unusual neurological symptoms. This led to a conversation about the rarest condition I had ever seen. A couple of the other doctors joined in. Everyone was enthusiastic to talk about this.

Apart from these moments of odd joy, the week was hard work. I felt that many people, both staff and patients, were looking at my appearance. Two people approached me to ask if I was okay. One was my friend and colleague, Lucy, who told me that I really didn't look well. I felt relief that I was able to say that I had made a GP appointment; not just relief that I had done so, but relief that it didn't look like I hadn't noticed myself. I was embarrassed by the idea that I hadn't noticed how odd I looked and had only just done something about it.

My last shift was on Thursday evening. It was really difficult. I spent the last couple of hours counting down the minutes until I could go home. Thankfully, I was on with another consultant, and I let him do all the work. I felt guilty but I really couldn't do anything. I nearly said that I was going home early as I didn't feel well. But something inside me wanted to stay to the bitter end. It felt important.

The minute my shift was ended, I got up, with some difficulty and made my way into the office to get my stuff. I said goodbye to everyone and that I would see them next week and then I left. I picked my way through all the trolleys squeezed into the corridor — not an easy feat, given my size — and then out past all the ambulances waiting to offload. I hardly noticed them anymore, so common had the sight become.

## January 2023: Friday 13th

I only realised on the day of my GP appointment that it was Friday 13th. That doesn't bode well, I couldn't help thinking. I even wondered if that was a good enough reason to cancel it.

The walk to the surgery felt slightly surreal. I couldn't quite believe that I was doing this after avoiding it for so long. I wasn't sure what to say. I would have to tell the GP that I just kept putting on weight and no matter what I did I couldn't lose it, and that people had begun to say that there might be something else wrong with me and I should see a doctor. I realised that I felt stupid that people were telling me that I needed to see a doctor when I was a doctor. Maybe it made me seem like not a very good doctor. Worse, I didn't know if there was something wrong with me or if I was just fat. This was like some embarrassing version of a rock and a hard place.

I wasn't sure how I could explain that I had tried to make sense of it all, but I just couldn't. I didn't know what to say to him to enable him to make sense of it. Then it hit me: I didn't have to. That was his job. I didn't need to be the doctor, I just needed to be the patient. I felt an odd sense of relief.

I was also glad that my face and upper body looked emaciated, to use my mother's description. I hoped that he would see that and believe that I had really tried to lose weight. And I had really tried, I reminded myself.

Ironically, despite my shape and size, I felt very small and vulnerable. Finally, I understood that one of the reasons that I had put off going to see my GP was that I was scared that I was going to be told off for being fat. That was the first time that I caught a glimpse of how great my shame was.

I was a doctor, and I knew a lot of doctors. The idea that any of us would feel that anyone should feel like that was ridiculous. But in the great tangle of my feelings, I held both of these opposing thoughts and both were equally true to me. I tried to understand how this could be, but it was too confusing. And anyway, I had arrived; I was at the surgery. All I had to do was hand this whole mess over to someone else. And, said the little voice inside me, if anyone makes you feel bad, just write a complaint about them. You're an adult now; you don't have to take it. No-one has the right to make you feel bad.

As it happened, I had no cause to complain; the GP was absolutely lovely to me. He listened quietly as I told him the story. He only interjected once and that was when I told him how my shape had led people to think that I was pregnant.

'That must have been very distressing for you,' he said.

He said it in a way that made me feel that he genuinely meant it. And the strange thing was that, until he described my situation back to me as distressing, this had never occurred to me. I knew that I had felt distressed, but I had connected the distress to something that was my fault, namely my shape and my inability to lose weight. I had become lost in the idea that it was my responsibility and my responsibility alone to solve the problem.

He examined my belly and agreed that it didn't feel like typical ascites. He also weighed me. I felt the usual shame. I was shocked at my weight but not, surprisingly, because it was so much. I was overweight but not by nearly as much as I was expecting. I had weighed this much before at certain times of my life; in fact, I had been heavier at others. I thought of my skinny arms and legs and wondered quite how much — or how little — I would weigh without my belly.

'I think we need to refer you to be seen at the hospital,' he said. 'I will make a two-week-wait referral for you.'

I knew exactly what that meant.

'Do you think it's cancer, then?' I asked.

Before I had come into the surgery, I had suspected that I might be referred as a two-week-wait patient because of the strangeness of my symptoms, but hearing it was still a shock.

As a doctor, I know that in these situations you can be thinking one of two different things. You can either not know what something is, but you are aware that the first thing you need to exclude is cancer. Or you can look at someone and think, this is cancer.

I wanted to know which one he was thinking. I hated asking him the question, but I couldn't stop myself. It is a horrible question to have to answer. It's the kind of conversation that follows you home and can hang around with you for several days. And even when you do manage to force it out of your immediate thoughts, it lurks in the shadows, popping out to haunt you from time to time.

He had been so kind and empathetic to me, I wanted to be the same for him. I felt stupid asking the question. As a fellow doctor, I felt that I should know as much as he did.

But the difference was that I wanted the answer to be no, far more than he could want it to be. After all, I had created a whole other reality to live in to keep the answer being no and that world was being dismantled right in front of me. For a moment, I wanted him to collude with me and keep that world intact. I sensed, correctly, that he wouldn't. And by correctly, I mean that it would have been the wrong thing for him to do; and by correctly, I mean that my sense was right and he didn't.

'Look,' he said. 'I have done this for long enough now to know that you can never know the answer to that question. But I do think that this looks like more than normal weight gain. Also, warning bells have obviously been ringing for your mother and your colleagues. I think we need to get it checked out.'

He then asked me which hospital I would like to be referred to. The choice included the hospital where I worked. For all my career, I had always thought that if I was unwell, I would like to be seen somewhere else. I imagined that I would want a bit of anonymity if I needed treatment.

But I suddenly felt differently. The concern shown to me by my two co-workers was one of the things that changed my mind. I was scared and, somehow, being seen in my workplace felt safe. I knew that everyone would take really good care of me. I didn't doubt that I would be taken care of in other hospitals. But my own workplace felt like home and that's where I wanted to be.

He also said that he could either refer me to the gynae department or gastro as, if I did have abdominal distension, it could be from either an ovarian cause or something in my abdomen. Whenever I had read the words 'filthy great tumour', I had always thought of ovarian cancer. So, I said that I didn't mind, but maybe to start off with gynae.

Then I did something I had never done before in my career. I asked for time off work. I felt guilty, but I just didn't think I could cope any longer.

On the walk home from the surgery, I had to go up a very steep hill. On the way down, it had occurred to me that I would struggle to walk up it and so had thought out an alternative route. But when I got there, I took a deep breath and walked up as fast as I could. I didn't stop until I reached the top. See, I told myself, you can't have cancer. You couldn't possibly have walked all the way up that hill like that if you had cancer, could you?

## January 2023: Three Things

I went home to wait. Two weeks, said the little voice in my head. It was beginning to sound quite cheery.

The next morning, I went to get my bloods taken. It was at another hospital in the area. I arrived at 9:45. I had planned to go earlier, but a great weariness had come over me and I found it hard to leave the house.

The phlebotomy clinic was rammed, and the receptionist told me that she could only give me an appointment in an hour and a half's time.

I sat in the hospital café with my Kindle. I was half-reading, half-watching everyone else. A couple of doctors were ordering coffee. A bleep went off and one of them gave the weary sigh of someone having to work the weekend. It occurred to me that I wasn't there as a doctor but as a patient. It felt strange. It hit me that, if something was wrong with me, this might be my life for the foreseeable future.

I thought of the receptionist back at the phlebotomy clinic. One thing I had going for me in my new role as a patient was that when I was anxious, I had no desire to try and gain control of the situation. That's how lots of people deal with stress, but when I was stressed, all I wanted to do was connect with the people around me. It occurred to me that this was going to help me in whatever was going to happen next. I decided there and then that the more stressed I felt, the more I would try and connect with people around me. I found this comforting.

I tried to think of other things that might help me. I loved reading. Put me anywhere and I am happy as long as I have a book. So, I should look on this time as an opportunity to catch up on all the books on my Kindle.

I tried to think of a third thing. There is something about having things in threes. It is the number that appears over and over again in fairy tales, after all. I glanced down at my hand and the massive great veins on it. I would be relatively easy to take blood from and insert intravenous lines into. I ran through these three things in my head. No matter what was going to happen, I would try to focus on them.

On the way home, it suddenly occurred to me that maybe I didn't need to diet any more. Even if I did, surely I deserved something nice? I have often thought that one way of judging the strictness of any diet I was following was to look at what I considered a treat. That day when I went into the supermarket to get a treat, I bought myself bread and grapes.

## January 2023: It's Not the Waiting

It felt strange on the Monday morning to wake up and not have to go to work. It felt like I was on holiday, except, of course, that I wasn't.

I met a friend from work, Elisha, for lunch. As I walked down to meet her, I felt guilty, like I was 'pulling a sickie.' How embarrassing if this all turns out to be just weight gain, I thought. Getting time off work was worse than having people give up their seats for me on the tube because they thought that I was close to giving birth.

Elisha was worried about me. I told her that I didn't think it could be that serious. If anything, I felt better that day. Perhaps it was not having to be at work that was making me feel brighter. A lot of my problems could be related to the conditions in which we were now expected to do our jobs. She agreed with me, but I knew she was doubtful. I felt the world that I had crafted to live in since October break down a little bit more.

The next day, the GP phoned with my blood results. Firstly, the CA125 was normal. CA125, if raised, indicates ovarian cancer. When I was told that mine wasn't raised, I felt the same way I used to feel when I found out that I had passed an exam. I had thought it unlikely that I could be walking around with ovarian cancer and a large effusion for eight months, and I had been right. I had just allowed myself to get worked up into a state.

However, a couple of my blood tests were abnormal. My haemoglobin was low, signifying anaemia. That could explain the severe tiredness.

In some ways, I was relieved that my bloods were abnormal; it seemed to justify not being at work. But I was unnerved, too.

As my CA125 was normal, my GP referred me to the gastro department. I was back in the strange limbo of waiting. Waiting is the hardest part, a few people said to me. It is said so often that it has become accepted wisdom. For me, it wasn't true. I had never thought waiting was the hardest part, and it was still the finding out that I hated more.

At least I could still write. Writing was the one thing that I loved that my shape had not taken from me. Since the start of the pandemic, I had written every day. Over the last few months, it had been the only pleasure that I had. It transported me to a better place. And now it also brought structure to my day.

I was working on a strange little children's story. It had started off as a bit of a joke. One night, in my writing group, I had created the character of an evil robin. I couldn't get the idea out of my head. I had then started seeing robins everywhere. It was December, so that was hardly a surprise, but I took it as a sign and decided to write about him.

In the story, the villain, Jack Frost, has kidnapped the robin and is overfeeding him on bad pennies and spoilt broth so that he will become bloated up with badness. By the end, the robin is enormous. Although it reads like a children's story, there is a darkness to it. Of course, that is the way with many children's stories. It felt to me like it came from somewhere deep in my subconscious. There was something wild and chaotic about it. I can't explain this except to say that, to me, it felt as though it had a jagged quality to it. I assumed that, in amongst all the chaos, it was trying to say something to me about my working conditions.

## January 2023: A Day of Firsts

Now that I was off work, waiting, time seemed to run differently, as if it had warped. On the Thursday, six days after I saw my GP, I went up to the hospital to see one of the gastroenterology consultants, Dr Dariush Sadigh. Normally, I went in through the Emergency Department entrance, but that day, I used the main entrance, arriving in a different and unfamiliar space. The hospital was like two different worlds superimposed on each other.

I made my way to a part of the hospital I didn't really know. Navigating it felt difficult — and I was someone who was comfortable being in a hospital. Suddenly, I understood why even stepping into one would add a layer of stress to being a patient or relative. For many people, a hospital must seem like a foreign country with its own sounds, smells and incomprehensible place names. I told Dariush the whole story. I felt silly telling him, as he was someone I knew professionally but, just like the GP, he was lovely to me.

Dariush asked if I had lost my appetite. This was quite complex. Yes, I didn't want to eat much but that was intentional. I was on a diet, after all, and surely that is the silver bullet of many diets: the idea that you may feel hungry to begin with but then your body adjusts.

Not wanting to eat is good, isn't it? It's what many people are aiming for. Being told that you have a big appetite always sound like a criticism. No-one ever describes themselves as having a 'small appetite'. They just say, airily, that they never eat breakfast or lunch. They make a virtue out of forgetting to stop and have a meal. Somehow, wanting to eat is a weakness. How I had longed to have a small appetite, or not to have a big one. Not to enjoy food quite as much as I did. Not to think of it as one of life's great pleasures and be constantly looking forward to my next meal. I had spent my life longing to be one of those people who have a *laissez faire* attitude to eating. But now that I was, I wasn't enjoying it nearly as much as I thought I would. And now I was explaining this to a doctor and I knew the reason that he was asking was that it's a big red flag for cancer.

Finally, he asked if I felt tired. We both started to laugh.

'Of course you are,' he said. 'You're an Emergency Medicine consultant.'

Dariush sent me for a CT scan. The plan was that, afterwards, I would go to the Day Treatment Centre, for an iron transfusion to treat my anaemia. Dariush would come to speak to me there and, if the scan showed fluid, he would aspirate some. I waited for my CT in an area of the hospital where I had sent numerous people but had never actually been myself. I had never had a CT either. It was definitely a day of firsts in my new life as a patient.

By the time I went to the Day Treatment Centre, it was late afternoon and the ward was emptying out. As I lay and waited, I listened to the usual sounds of a hospital ward: a patient being given their discharge instructions, the scrape of a chair, the sound of curtains being opened, muffled conversation, the occasional burst of laughter.

Someone came and started my infusion. I got out my Kindle and tried to read. Point number two in my list was 'now you have time to read all the books on your Kindle.' But I was only half-concentrating. I kept on having to read the same thing over and over again.

Then I heard another familiar sound: as familiar as a kettle coming to the boil or the traffic on the Holloway Road. So common that, most of the time, I don't know if I even pick it out specifically. It's just another note in the backing track of my life. But I heard it distinctly that afternoon. The sound a procedures trolley makes, as it's being wheeled across the floor.

Procedures trolleys are stainless steel trolleys holding equipment for a bedside procedure. They must be a distant relative of the shopping trolley, in that they always seem to be fighting to go in a different direction from the person pushing them.

## January 2023: The Moment

Months later, I spoke to a friend who is one of the clinical psychologists in the hospital. She asked me whether there was an exact moment when I accepted that I had cancer. Then she got me describe everything about that moment: what it felt like, both in my head and in my body, and any sounds or smells or other things that I noticed.

And that was the sound of that moment: the sound of the procedures trolley being wheeled towards me across the ward by Dariush. That is the sound that I associate with realising that I had cancer.

On the trolley were needles and syringes, local anaesthetic, specimen bottles, gauze swabs, sterile fluid, a dressing pack, all the paraphernalia he needed if he was going to aspirate something. And that something was me.

As soon as I heard and saw that trolley, it felt as if all the thoughts in my head dropped. Like in a cartoon, they all slipped from where they were held in my brain and ended up lying misshapen and floppy on the floor around me. And as I was frantically trying to pick them all up, Dariush was cleaning a small spot on my abdomen. I hardly felt the local anaesthetic go in.

I watched as my great big belly easily swallowed the green needle. And then, as he pulled back on the plunger, I watched in horrified fascination as the syringe filled up with fluid.

'Fuck me,' I thought. 'I've got ascites. That's why none of my dieting was working.'

I was full up with ascites, full to bursting with ascites. I had been walking around, going about my day-to-day life with a great big belly full of ascites. It had been there for — well, I don't know for how long — eight months, a year, maybe longer. It wasn't excess weight; it was ascites.

'Do you think that this could be cancer?' I asked, as I watched him squirt the fluid, my ascites, into a specimen jar. Inside my head, the doctor part of me rolled her eyes; she couldn't quite believe I was asking this question. Of course, he thinks you have cancer, she muttered.

But, to be honest, the doctor part of me wasn't particularly dominant at that moment. Small parts of my brain were breaking into panic, small islands of terror, but most of it just sat there, lumpen, and frozen.

My conscious mind had a lot to deal with. It needed to recalibrate everything it had believed to be true about the last year. I replayed people asking me if I was pregnant, and I tried to add the new information that no, I had ascites and probably cancer.

But beyond that, I had a sense that my subconscious wasn't that surprised. It was as if it had known and the rest of me was just catching up. Finally, I could see that it had recognised that something was going on for quite some time. I was both the first and the last person to realise that there was something seriously wrong with me. While I ignored it, it wasn't fully real. But now, by acknowledging it, I had brought it into being. I couldn't avoid it anymore.

I couldn't really believe that I had been walking round with ascites for all that time. I couldn't believe that there was something wrong with me; more than that, that something had gone so wrong inside me that I was producing all that fluid.

As a doctor, you are taught to take a history and ask for symptoms and then examine the patient and look for clinical signs. Now, we've all had experience of having symptoms of something, so, hearing a patient describe a symptom (even if it is one that you have never experienced), is still something you can identify with. But signs are different; signs are rarer. People take pictures of them for textbooks and bring medical students in to see them. It's a figure of speech to say 'people would pay good money for...' but I wouldn't be surprised to hear that trainee doctors might be happy to pay something to see a patient with a good clinical sign in those desperate days leading up to any medical exam. Doctors would certainly come in on their days off if there was anyone on a ward with one.

And I had been walking around with one, dragging it about with me all that time and had not even realised. I was the medical equivalent of the people who go on the *Antiques Roadshow* with some type of receptacle that they use to keep their keys in, only to discover that it is a Lalique bowl. Something had gone so wrong with me that I had an actual clinical sign: a florid clinical sign, as the textbooks would describe it; a florid clinical sign, but no symptoms. It was all very confusing.

And, more than that, it was most likely to be cancer. I knew that and Dariush knew that. I was a person with cancer. I couldn't grasp it.

Dariush told me that, at present, all they could see on my scan was lots of fluid. There was no other obvious clue as to what was causing it. Everything else looked normal, including my liver. I was to come back the next day to the radiology department and they would take samples for biopsy under ultrasound guidance. They would also insert a drain to remove as much of the fluid as possible, which would make me feel better.

Dariush asked me what I was going to do that evening. When I told him I was going home by myself, he was worried, and suggested I phone my friend, Lucy. Lucy told me to get a taxi to her house.

I stood at the main entrance trying not to lose my composure. The rest of the world moved round me or, in the case of the traffic, didn't move, as if nothing had happened. And, in the grand scheme of things, nothing had happened to the rest of the world. It was only to me and my world that something had happened. As I stood there waiting, I wondered how many people I had walked past in my position, just walked past on my way home, angry about something that had happened during the day or thinking about something really banal like what I was going to have for tea.

## January 2023: A Remarkable Conversation

The next morning, I got up in time to do my writing before I went to the hospital. It felt incredibly important to me that I made sure that I wrote. Maybe it was because it was a part of me that I still had. Or perhaps focusing on writing was strong enough to stop all the other thoughts. And though it was only for a short while, that helped.

I got the bus to the hospital. During the previous year, no matter how exhausted I had felt, I always made myself climb the stairs and sit on the top deck. Firstly, I was scared that if there were no seats downstairs, someone would offer me theirs. Secondly, I had always sat on the top deck. I was worried that, if I found an excuse not to climb the stairs, I would get out of the habit. And then one day I would discover that I could no longer do it. But on that morning, I decided that I would treat myself and stay downstairs. So what if someone offered me their seat? I might not be pregnant, but I did have cancer. Somehow it didn't seem quite so humiliating, now that there was something actually wrong with me. And let's face it no-one could argue that there wasn't. No-one argues with cancer.

I was seen by an interventional radiologist, Dr Jeevan Kumaradevan. He was going to use USS guidance to take biopsies and then put in a drain to remove the ascites. Jeevan was yet another person who was so lovely to me, he almost made me cry. I can't remember exactly what he said; it was something like he was so sorry that I was having to experience this, but at least now we could get a diagnosis and I could start receiving the correct treatment for it.

He began by taking biopsies from my omentum. I hadn't thought about the omentum since medical school. I remember it being described, rather unpleasantly, as a fatty apron that hangs over the abdominal cavity. It popped into my head that it was also called the abdominal policeman. It had something to do with fighting infection. The biopsy itself was painless. I began to relax a bit.

Then Jeevan put a drain into my belly to get rid of some of the fluid. I would hesitate to use the term 'looking forward to this' but I had been pleased at the idea of losing some of it. Would the fluid shoot out at high pressure? Would my belly deflate like a balloon? And what I would look like without it?

The drain went in easily.

Nothing came out.

I watched Jeevan as he concentrated. Using the ultrasound machine for guidance, he manipulated the position of the drain. It made no difference. Finally, he removed it and tried with a bigger tube. Still no fluid came.

He took a big syringe and a needle and inserted that, instead. I could see him struggle with the plunger on the syringe; there was some kind of resistance. Finally, he withdrew a thick, viscous-like substance. It reminded me of glue. I knew about ascites but not thick ascites. Not ascites that was too thick to drain. I had never heard about this before. I didn't understand it. There was something alien about it; it looked like ectoplasm and it was inside me. I started to panic.

Then Dariush appeared. He might have said 'Knock, knock' outside the curtains. Doctors often say this if they are going to open closed curtains.

Jeevan was decanting the ectoplasm into specimen pots. He couldn't drain my belly. We were still going to be in this together for the time being.

Dariush pulled up a seat. He explained that another of the radiology consultants had looked at my scan. She thought that there was something in my left ovary. It looked like I had ovarian cancer. Dariush thought that this was likely. In his experience, I looked too well for someone with a cancer of the gastrointestinal tract. When he had done the blood tests yesterday, he had also checked for another tumour marker called CEA. It was elevated at 1400. I didn't know the normal range, but I had a suspicion that 1400 was very high. The specimens would be sent for analyses. My case would be discussed at the big gynae malignancy team meeting the next Wednesday.

I understood these words and terms, but they were difficult to take in when applied to me. Anyway, there was only one question I wanted to ask.

'Am I going to die from this?'

Yet again, I knew that this was a ridiculous question. I even knew the answer, which was 'no-one knows, but probably.' I have had to answer that question on a few occasions; I was very aware that I was now making another doctor answer it for me.

Dariush was so kind. He told me that he didn't know what was going to happen but, in his experience, people frequently said that, in the end, they always felt better for a diagnosis. What I was going to go through wouldn't be easy, but it might be better than what I had already been through.

I left the radiology department in a daze and went down to the coffee area. I called Lucy and she came down immediately.

'Why was the ascites so thick?' she asked.

I didn't really know, I shrugged.

'Okay,' she said. 'What do you need me to do to help you?'

I asked whether, if I had to have an operation, as I was sure that I would, I could go and stay with her for a few days after I got out of hospital. This was something that I had been trying not to think about, but it had been bothering me since my GP had referred me. I could now see that it had been bothering me for longer than that. It was probably one of the things that was fuelling my denial. I lived alone and had no family in London. I didn't see how it was possible that I could cope with being sick, so sick that I might need looking after, when I had no-one to look after me. Illness wasn't just affecting my body; now my whole lifestyle seemed precarious.

'Of course,' she said. 'In fact, if you wanted to, you could move in now.'

The relief was immeasurable. I didn't need or want to do that, but it made things easier just knowing that I could. The relief was so great that

I began to feel marginally better. I said something vaguely amusing that I would hesitate to call a joke. We both laughed at it much more than it deserved.

I was glad to find that I could still laugh. But there was something else too. To find that that part of me still existed, unchanged by everything, brought me some kind of reassurance. Despite everything that was going on, I was happy to discover that I still existed inside my head.

There was a power in being able to laugh. That feeling of power brought with it the faintest glimmer of hope. I don't know what that hope was based on. But, maybe, that is the nature of hope. It doesn't necessarily have to be based on anything — sometimes it just shows up.

'If I get through all this, when it's over, let's go away and treat ourselves,' I said. 'We will have a few days by the seaside.'

'Definitely,' Lucy replied.

Even suggesting it increased that sense of power and glimmer of hope. It takes a lot of bravery to dream and hope for the best. I was surprised to find it in myself that morning, as I have never thought of myself as a hopeful person. And, deep down, I fully expected that I was going to die. I suspected that Lucy thought the same thing. I later found out that she did. But neither of us said it. It was probably the most remarkable conversation that I have had in my entire life.

Lucy would be the first to describe herself as *not* a touchy-feely person but, as I left, she touched my arm. I will remember that gesture forever.

I couldn't face getting on the bus, so I walked home from the hospital. It felt strange to be walking when I was, perhaps, dying. The biggest irony was that, physically, I felt better than I had in ages. It must have been because I had had some time away from work and all the madness there.

## January 2023: The Important Stuff

I phoned my sister and my mother. I felt guilty for the pain I was causing. I asked my sister to contact my best friend Alison at home and tell her. I realised that I couldn't deal with other people's reactions.

Then I settled down to wait. Wait for what? Not two weeks, anymore. Wait to die? I couldn't get my head around that. I didn't feel like I was going to die. But then again, I had no idea what feeling like you were going to die was supposed to be like.

I don't really know what happened to that weekend. My only ambition for each day was to make sure I wrote a little. The rest of the time I just lay under my electric fleece in a daze.

I just couldn't believe that I had cancer. The only time in my life that I could equate this to was when my father had died. Then I couldn't believe that I had become one of those people who had lost a parent. And, now, I couldn't believe that I was one of those people who had cancer; I was a member of the cancer club. I said this to a friend. She said, of course I didn't believe it. No-one grows up dreaming that these things will happen to them. This is not how we imagine our lives when we are children.

I had always thought that doctors had such a dark sense of humour to deal with the suffering they saw around them. Now I understood that we hide something else in that darkness: the terror that one day this will be us.

On the Monday, I met Elisha for lunch. She told me about some new irritation at work. Suddenly, I became furious, really furious.

'Don't put up with it,' I said. 'Seriously, look at me as a cautionary tale.

Think of how much of my life I have given up to work, and for what? Just don't take it.'

It was a damp, drizzly sort of day. As I was walking home along the Holloway Road, I noticed a house. It had a wild, overgrown garden and in it was a spindly tree. The tree was tall — taller than the house — and right on top of it was perched a bird. Both the tree and the bird were swaying in the breeze. I thought that it was one of the most beautiful things that I had ever seen. It was like something from a Japanese painting. It had an elegance about it, like a haiku brought to life. It seemed perfect to me. I was transfixed by it.

Every time I tried to walk on, I couldn't. I just couldn't tear myself away from watching that bird balanced on top of the tree. It struck me that now my life was running out, I had all the time in the world to look at things like this. Now, it seemed to me that that bird on the tree was the important stuff of life. Stuff I hadn't paid enough attention to before.

On the Tuesday morning, I had an MRI scan. I got up early to make sure that I could write before I went to it.

On the bus, I treated myself to sitting downstairs again. You had better be careful, I told myself. See how easily this is becoming a habit. Who cares? If I'm going to die, who cares?' said another voice in my head.

At the MRI scanner, a nurse took my details and inserted an intravenous cannula. I really didn't like being in the scanner. I felt that I only just managed to squeeze my huge belly in. I felt like an animal in a trap; like I was being forced further and further into a tunnel, a tunnel with no light at the end.

When it was over, the nurse that had inserted my cannula came up to me. 'I didn't realise it was you,' she said. We were both wearing masks and she pulled hers down. I recognised her as one of the nurses from the Acute Admissions Ward.

'I'm up here now,' she said. 'How are you?'

'I've got all of this going on,' I said. 'It's a bit of a worry.'

She pulled me in and gave me a big hug. I stood there, enjoying the warmth and closeness of it.

Afterwards, I walked home. Dying or not, I did not want to get out of the habit of that. On the way, I stopped at a café for a cup of coffee. I remembered that I didn't need to diet anymore and decided to treat myself to a cake, except they didn't have anything that I wanted.

As I sat drinking my coffee, I realised that something was making me feel a bit better, a bit more cheerful. It took a while to figure out that it was the hug. I had really liked being hugged. Over the last year, I had been shutting more and more people out. I had built a fortress round myself as I was terrified of letting anyone in, in case they asked me if I was pregnant.

And, oh, how I had hated having to live that way. But now I didn't have to keep people out anymore. I might be dying but at least now I could connect with people again. And living a life without connecting to others is not really a life at all; at least, not to me. I felt a little happier at that.

Perhaps there was the faintest glimmer of light at the end of the tunnel after all.

## January 2023: Choices and Transitions

When I got home, I spoke to my friend, Sue, a clinical psychologist at the hospital. I told her that I felt a real reluctance to get out of bed in the morning. But then, at night, I felt the same reluctance to get off the sofa and go to bed. To me, there was something more to this than just the physical disinclination; I felt that there was a psychological component to it.

She agreed, and said that maybe it was something that we could work with. It seemed to show that once I was somewhere, I could adapt to being there and feel comfortable; it was the transitions that I struggled with. I should remind myself of this every time I had to make one.

After we hung up, I started to think about the music I wanted at my funeral. I decided on the hymns *Dear Lord and Father of Mankind,* which had always been my favourite at school, and *Abide with Me,* which is, apparently, popular at funerals. My love for it came from the time I heard it in Preston, after my father's death. It was a Sunday, and I was due to start work at eight, and so my alarm went off at seven. I had an old-fashioned radio alarm clock, tuned to Radio Two. It was one of those September days when you realise that summer is definitely over, and autumn has arrived. The summer in which my father had died had passed; time was moving on.

His death was still recent, but the initial rawness of it was healing over. I was settling into a routine; learning how to live my life without him. But, in a way, moving on seemed a betrayal of sorts. Moving on required letting go and I didn't want to do that. I wanted to hold onto him.

I could see through the curtains that it was a dismal, grey day. Like one of those games where you use the weather to describe your mood, I felt dismal and grey too. I didn't want to get up for work. I thought of all those boring childhood Sundays: my mother making the dinner, my father reading the papers. A world I'd longed to escape from. And now that world was gone, and it would never be back. I would never see my father again.

Then the radio played a choir singing *Abide with Me*. I thought it was one of the most beautiful things I had ever heard, and I just lay there with my eyes closed, listening to it. I started to cry, but it was as if the music lifted me up and carried me along with it. It comforted me and swept me into the day. I remember there and then thinking, when I die, I want this played at my funeral. Then I got up and got ready to go into work.

So that was the hymns decided. Then there would be the final flourish, the piece of music that your coffin will be carried out to: your last chance to stamp your personality on the world. I had discussed this several times, over the years, with different sets of friends. It was one of those conversations like what would your last meal on earth be.

My choice has varied down the ages. But my present one was The Waterboys singing *The Whole of the Moon*. It occurred to me that the lyrics could imply that I thought about myself in a slightly grandiose manner, but if there's one time when you can get away with being grandiose about yourself, surely it's when you're dead. Also, there was an added poignancy as it was often the last song of the night in Kelly's Nightclub in Portrush back in the days when I spent a lot of time there. Or was it? I couldn't remember for sure. They played *Celebrate [This Party's Over, I'm Going Home]* too. There would be a certain irony in using that.

Or maybe I should go out in one final, spine-tingling blaze of glory and punk rock anarchy with the Undertones and *Teenage Kicks*, a song that I can't hear without feeling a rush of excitement. And then it hit me: I'd be dead. This wasn't just some silly conversation in the pub. I'd actually be dead. I'd no longer exist. I would never hear *Teenage Kicks* again.

For a moment, I thought of playing it, but I couldn't bear it. I couldn't bear hearing it knowing that it could be the last time I would ever hear it. And even if it wasn't, my life was on a countdown now; anything could be the last time. And what about all the other songs that I might never hear again? Ella Fitzgerald singing *Every Time We Say Goodbye*; The Human League and *Don't You Want Me*; The Cure and *Friday I'm in Love*; the Pet Shop Boys *Always on My Mind*; Julie London and *Fly Me to the Moon*. Songs came filling my head thick and fast. A whole lifetime's worth. How long would I need in order to hear them all, one last time?

It was as if each song was attached to a thread, which if you gave it a little tug, pulled down a memory: sitting, three to a seat, on the school bus; going to university; the wonderful feeling of falling in love; the first time that I went on holiday with friends.

Perceived wisdom has it that when you think you're going to die, you regret all the things that you never did. But I didn't really care that I had never seen the Pyramids or the Taj Mahal. What I couldn't bear was the loss of all the tiny, ordinary little things — little things that I hardly even noticed or thought about half the time. Life is like a story, and I wouldn't be in it anymore. It would go on without me and I would never find out what happens next.

Suddenly, I began to panic; I couldn't bear it. Then I thought of the bird balanced on the tree, swaying in the breeze. I began to calm down a little.

I realised that, at least, I had had a good life. Not everything had turned out the way I had wanted, but when does it ever? No-one gets that. But what I had got had brought me mostly joy. And as for the bad parts, the majority no longer seemed important. I felt a huge sense of relief that I didn't have children. I had an inkling of how unbearable that must feel for anyone in my position. I sat for a little longer and let myself calm down until I was able to go and make myself a cup of coffee.

## January 2023: Four Things

On the Wednesday, I found it extra hard to get out of bed. There were four things that I had to do, four unpleasant things, and I really didn't want to do any of them. Even the thought of having to perform the simplest of tasks now exhausted me.

These tasks were: to check my blood pressure, wash my hair, pay my tax bill and find out what was to happen next with regard to my cancer.

As well as everything else, my GP had noticed that my blood pressure was high. He had suggested that I buy a machine and check it twice a day for a week. I filed the results online and he would decide if I needed treatment. I hated doing this, and the pressure remained high, which made me feel bad. I wasn't worried about it being high; it just made me feel like a failure.

My tax bill had been calculated several months earlier. I just hadn't got round to paying it and the deadline was approaching. I paid it online each year and from memory there was always something that I found difficult in doing so, but I couldn't remember what. The very thought of doing it was sending me into a spin.

As for my hair, the very idea of getting my broken shower fixed was beyond anything that I was currently able to manage. This meant washing my hair with a jug of water, which was highly unpleasant.

Finally, I had to find out about my treatment.

Dariush Sadigh had told me that my scans would be discussed at an MDT meeting that morning with the gynaecology/oncology team. They would review my case and all my results and decide what to do next. I was pretty sure Dariush had said he would phone me and let me know. But I had this tiny bit of doubt as to whether I was supposed to be phoning him.

I forced myself out of bed, and took up my downstairs position under my fleecy, electric blanket. I did my writing and then lay there trying to force myself to complete my tasks. Finally, partly motivated by my desire to have a cup of coffee, I took my blood pressure. I wasn't supposed to check it if I had recently drunk coffee. It was still high.

My laptop was right beside me, so I registered my readings, and then logged in and paid my tax bill. Whatever it was that had confused me previously didn't seem to confuse me this time and I completed the whole thing without much problem.

Next was my hair. The whole process was made even more dismal as my flat was freezing. Due to all the problems with soaring energy prices, I was trying not to turn on my heating. That was one of the reasons I spent most of my time under my fleecy, electric blanket. Suddenly it struck me: if I was going to die, did it really matter how high my gas bill was? Turn the heating on, I told myself; turn the place into a greenhouse, why don't you? It won't really matter much if you're going to be dead.

After I managed to wash my hair, I treated myself to a piece of toast. It was lunchtime and I was exhausted. It had taken me all morning to complete three simple tasks. A fortnight earlier I had been able to run an emergency department.

But the fourth task still remained. I sat for a while and waited. Finally, I decided that I would phone. Dariush answered on the third ring.

'I was just about to phone you,' he said. 'Now, would you like me to tell you on the phone or would you rather come in and we can talk face-to-face.'

'Just tell me now,' I replied.

Even me, Little Miss It's-Not-The-Waiting-It's-The-Finding-Out, just wanted to know now.

'Your results are back, and it looks like pseudomyxoma peritonei.'

Hold the wagon. Incongruously, that was the first thing that popped into my head when I heard my diagnosis. 'Hold the wagon' is not a phrase

I had ever used or even thought about using before and, nor, apart from writing this, have I found myself using again. But there it was in my head.

To be fair to my brain, there was a huge amount of chaos going on in there. Part of it, the part that had been busy preparing itself for the news that I had ovarian cancer was flummoxed. It had been sitting primed and ready for the news; waiting in anticipation to have to accept it as reality instead of supposition; expecting simultaneously to be taking it in and processing what was to happen next, formulating a plan of how I was going to manage and, perhaps, hearing some timelines around death. The death timeframe was important as it influenced location of death, either London or home. And now that part of my brain was sitting there idle, gradually accepting that it might not be needed after all.

Meanwhile, another part of my brain was screaming, 'So it's not ovarian cancer then?' Yet another bit was muttering, 'What the fuck is pseudomyxoma peritonei?' But even as it was doing so, from deep within my head, in the part where distant memory is stored, something was creakily coming to life. Ancient wheels and cogs were turning.

There was something familiar about that name, but from where? How did I know it? Then I had an image in my head: a list of conditions, numbered A-E, all typed out neatly in small print. Pseudomyxoma peritonei was one of them. Now, where had I seen that before? And then I had it: it was my old foe from all those years ago: the old MRCP Part 1 exam.

## January 2023: One in a Million

Pseudomyxoma peritonei, as I was to learn that afternoon and over the next few weeks, is a very rare condition. It occurs in about 1 in 1,000,000 people. That's why it was always popping up in the exam, with its fondness for the obscure. I had done well to remember anything about it at all. Many of my doctor friends had never heard of it or, if they had, had now forgotten it.

Not only is it rare, it is also rather peculiar. It is generally caused by an isolated mucinous tumour of the appendix, which ruptures. This fills the abdominal cavity with lots of cells which invade the peritoneum, the thin lining that covers the inside of the abdominal cavity and the organs that lie inside it. The cells of the peritoneum then produce a mucous-like fluid. This was why my ascites was so thick.

Even rarer, though, are cases where it is not caused by a ruptured tumour of the appendix. In some, it may be caused by a ruptured dermoid cyst. Dermoid cysts, or teratomas, form on the ovaries. They can grow very large and — in some cases — hair, bone or teeth will grow inside them. I was a little bit obsessed with them when I learned about them at medical school. There was something grotesquely fascinating about the pictures showing clumps of hair tangled up with isolated teeth and shards of bone. They didn't seem real; more like something from a horror story. My appendix looked normal on my scans, but there was something in my left ovary, and so the suspicion was that mine might have developed in that way.

On the positive side, as pseudomyxoma spreads through the peritoneum, it will always be contained in the abdominal cavity. However, the build-up of the thick, mucous-like fluid will eventually compress the organs, causing all sorts of problems such as an obstruction of the small bowel. And it can be fatal. I later discovered that it was what had killed Audrey Hepburn.

It is so rare that it is managed by only two centres in the country: Basingstoke and Manchester. Dariush had referred me to Basingstoke. I didn't even know where Basingstoke was. The treatment is an operation and local chemotherapy: chemo put directly into the abdominal cavity at the time of the surgery.

I have described myself as being stunned on a few occasions in my life. I now realise that I never had been. Because after that phone call, I was genuinely stunned. I just sat there and then I started — well, I don't know what I started doing. Even whilst I was doing it, I couldn't figure out whether I was laughing or crying. Tears were streaming down my face, my nose was running, and my body was shaking and convulsing.

I couldn't completely adjust to the new reality. The most recent reality had been difficult enough, but this was a whole different ball game. I was suffering from a disease that was so rare that I was now one in a million and that was not just a figure of speech. But, on the positive side, I didn't have ovarian cancer. Maybe I wasn't going to die after all.

Some people may find it strange, but I was almost giddy with joy when I found out that I had pseudomyxoma peritonei; certainly, I was giddy with relief that I didn't have ovarian cancer. From everything I had read, having ovarian cancer with a huge effusion like mine had an extremely poor prognosis. To be honest, the prognosis appeared to be death. And I had been delivered from it by a million-to-one shot. I couldn't quite get my head around it. It was like something from a book or one of those made-for-TV movies that you watch when you are off work sick.

I had an illness that I had never encountered in my 28-year career. A lot of Emergency Medicine is pattern recognition and I had never encountered this pattern before. It was a condition for which I had no mental blueprint.

Neither had most of my doctor friends. Not just the Emergency Medicine physicians; hardly anyone had heard of it.

That evening, after my diagnosis, I went to Lucy's for dinner. As I stood waiting for my taxi, I remembered trying to call a taxi outside the hospital when I had just found out that I had ascites. It was less than a week ago. Normal time seemed to have vanished and I was living in my own time zone. When the taxi arrived, the driver asked me what sort of a day I had had, was it alright?

'Yes, fine,' I replied.

I wanted to say, 'You have absolutely no idea. I thought that I had ovarian cancer and was going to die, but now I've found out that I have another type of cancer. It's very rare but I might not die after all.'

This was the thing. I had reached a point where I didn't have ovarian cancer, but I still didn't really know what my chances were. Now, at this point, many people might have started frantically googling. But I didn't; I preferred not to know. Perhaps it was denial again. Or just another version of 'it's not the waiting I don't like, it's the finding out.' Looking back, I just think I couldn't take anymore. It was all too much after the slow, insidious creep of illness over the previous year, followed by the shock and terror of the last days. I just wanted to be not scared for a while.

Over the next few days, I got up each morning and wrote. And I must have gone out to buy milk and bread at some point. I may have tried to watch some gentle TV: programmes like *Poirot* that I had seen countless times before, where I didn't even have to focus my frazzled brain on trying to follow a plot. Or I listened to podcasts. It was soothing to lie with my eyes closed, listening to other people having a conversation.

But, most of the time, I just lay under my electric fleece with my brain in the equivalent of hibernation mode. I didn't want to know what my chances of dying from this new, bizarre cancer were.

## January 2023: Not A Walk in the Park

I was pulled out of hibernation the following Tuesday, when I was phoned by a consultant surgeon from the Peritoneal Malignancy Unit in Basingstoke. I might have accepted my condition, but I didn't like hearing another doctor refer to 'your cancer'.

I was taught in medical school that patients retain very little of what you say to them. This is particularly true if what you are saying is shocking or frightening. I knew this, but I was still taken aback by how little of the conversation I remembered. The surgeon sent me an email a short time later, detailing what had been said, and I had no recollection of half of it.

Basically, I had pseudomyxoma peritonei and it appeared advanced. The fact that my CEA tumour marker was so high indicated that the tumour was aggressive, or had been there for a long time, or both. I have often used the word aggressive to describe tumours, but now it was my cancer, something that had taken up residence inside me, I found the word unnerving. It made me think of dogs. It was as if I had an angry dog inside me; something like a Pit Bull. If I was to have anything, I would much rather have something soft, like a Labrador or a Poodle.

I would need an operation. They would scrape away the lining, and my uterus, ovaries, appendix, spleen and other organs might all have to be removed. They would put in hyperthermic chemotherapy, and leave it for a while, and then rinse it out. The operation itself would take about ten hours; afterwards, I would go first to Intensive Care and then to the ward. I should expect to spend at least three weeks in hospital.

I was really freaked out at the idea of Intensive Care. Less than three weeks earlier, I had never even had an intravenous cannula inserted and now I was going to be in Intensive Care.

Worse, they might not be able to remove all the cancerous lining. This was most likely if it had settled on the small bowel. It might be too stuck down. They would remove what they could but some would have to stay, as they would have to leave the small bowel. They would take out my large bowel and I would have an ileostomy: a stoma immediately after my small bowel. Alternatively, they might get it all out, but have to remove some of my large bowel and give me a colostomy: a stoma at a different position

After I read all this, I was back in a world of terror again. For the last few days, I had just been so relieved that I did not have ovarian cancer that I hadn't thought about anything else. Now it looked like pseudomyxoma peritonei was not going to be a walk in the park either. And so I found myself asking another doctor if I might die.

He explained that the disease was so rare that it was hard to have accurate figures. However, if they got it all out, the five-year survival rate was 80%, and if they didn't, it was 30%. At least, I think that is what he said. I never googled it. I just found it too frightening.

Also, lots of other variables came in to play, such as how aggressive the tumour was (angry dog versus gentle dog) and my general condition before the operation. In the end, he couldn't tell me how much he would be able to remove until he opened me up. I was on the waiting list and would be contacted as soon as possible.

Finally, I asked whether there was any possibility, in all of this, that I might be able to go back to my normal life.

'Yes,' he said. 'Yes, there is.' It would take time, but many people said that at around three months, they began to feel their normal selves again.

I phoned my sister to tell her that pseudomyxoma peritonei might not be quite the walk in the park that I had hoped it would be.

'I know,' she said.

Whilst my brain had been hibernating, Sarah had googled every website she could find on the subject. She was relieved that I seemed to be coming up to speed with her. She was a real expert on the condition and was even referring to it as PMP. As I was too scared to start to read anything about it, we agreed that she would be the expert and the first port of call if I had any queries.

Next, I phoned and broke the news to my mother.

'I know,' she replied.

'How?'

'It's what Elizabeth's sister died of.'

'What?' I was bewildered. 'Who's Elizabeth and who was her sister?'

'Remember that book...?'

When I had been home in October, my mum had left, by my bed, a book which she thought I might like to look at. It was called *Light and Shade* and was a compilation of photographs that had been taken by a woman who had died of cancer. She was the sister of a friend of my mother's. I hadn't got round to looking at it. But it transpired that, when I was already unknowingly suffering from a rare, 'one in a million' type of cancer, my mother had given me a book compiled by someone else who had the same 'one in a million' type of cancer. What were the chances of that?

The truth was, now that I understood more about my pseudomyxoma peritonei, I was, in many ways, more scared than I had been when I thought that I had ovarian cancer. This was partly because the ovarian cancer had remained abstract, whereas now I had solid facts about pseudomyxoma peritonei. But there was more to it than that. With the ovarian cancer, there had always been a feeling of unreality; I couldn't grasp that I was a person that was soon going to die. This had actually been based on some degree of fact. Anyone with an ovarian tumour and an effusion is very unwell. And by very unwell, I mean sick and frail. I wasn't. Of course, I wasn't in great shape, but I was up and about. I was walking to my hospital appointments.

On some level, my story just didn't make any sense. Even Dariush, the gastroenterologist at the Whittington, had commented several times, in surprise, that I looked so well. It was like that part of a crime story when someone comes up with an explanation, but doesn't use all the clues.

But now that I knew what was going on, everything fitted together. I had gradually been accumulating a thick mucus-like substance over an unknown period of time. It explained my shape and why my belly was so hard. It made sense of everything that I had experienced the previous year.

And if it wasn't stopped, it would go on accumulating until it damaged my internal organs. At some point, it would be fatal. I had no idea of the timeframes around this and I didn't want to know. I just focused on the next step, which was the operation. And what an operation it would be. I later found out that its nickname is the 'mother of all operations'.

All I had was hope. And I had a very difficult relationship with hope. I hated having to rely on it. If they didn't get it all out, what then? I would have to live with some of the cancer still inside me. How long I might have in that case was another mystery, as was the quality of life I could expect. I would have a stoma, the idea of which appalled me.

I decided that, if they couldn't get it all out, I was going to go back home and live in Ireland. I wanted to be home and near my family. If they didn't get it out, there was no way I was continuing with my job. I had no idea if I would be left in a state where I would be able to work but, even if I was, I wasn't spending however long I had left struggling in my job anymore. My race was run, as far as Emergency Medicine was concerned.

What if I died under the anaesthetic or suffered major complications? Suddenly I was furious. I had had to go through the whole ovarian cancer terror and it had been such a relief when that had stopped. But now I was having to deal with this. I felt foolish, embarrassed now at my previous optimism. My diagnosis had delivered me from ovarian cancer. But delivered me to what?

## February 2023: Slipping Out of View

On the Wednesday, a most unlikely saviour prevented me from dwelling too much on my present condition. I was to have a colonoscopy on the Thursday, to see if my appendix looked abnormal, and so I had to take the bowel prep, a strong laxative, to completely empty out my intestines. It made me feel quite strange and so I went to bed in the afternoon. I tried to read, but spent most of my time in a state between sleep and wakefulness. It was as if I were shutting everything down.

The next morning, when I got off the bus, I turned towards the main entrance of the hospital: the one I used because I was a patient. I looked back towards the Emergency Department entrance. It occurred to me that I might never use it again.

As I sat in the Day Treatment Centre waiting area, I saw a consultant colleague from another specialty. She was rushing past, a coffee in one hand, her phone in the other. I thought of the me that I had been for most of my life. I inhabited a very different space in the hospital now. I watched her go down the stairs. It was like watching my old life disappear from view.

In the end, my colonoscopy was not as bad as I had feared. Despite the large amount of fluid, they got a good look at my appendix, and it appeared normal. For a moment, I hoped that this meant that I did not have cancer. It wasn't rational, but I wasn't being very rational about things just then.

I spent the night at Lucy's house. The next morning, as she was taking me home, I waited in the car as she took her daughter into the breakfast club at her school. We were high up, and I had a view across London. Once upon a time, I would have dismissed the day as grey. Now I could see that it had a stark beauty to it, with a silvery softness behind the gloom. Below me, the city was waking up. To many people it was just another ordinary day at the end of an ordinary week. But to me, it was spectacular. How many more days like this had I got left?

When I got home, I found out that my operation had been scheduled for the following Thursday. I think that this was when I probably freaked out the most. It felt much too soon. The operation was going to be in London and not Basingstoke, as the team had an arrangement with one of the London hospitals. I phoned Sarah, and she started to make preparations to come over. She asked if she could stay at my flat, and I was horrified. I hadn't been able to do much for so long that it was in chaos. I was so embarrassed that she was going to see it. I thought about telling her not to come, but I really didn't know if I would be able to cope. Anyway, I knew that neither she nor my mother would even hear of such a thing.

I was terrified at the idea of the operation. I couldn't think of it without panicking. Finally, I told myself that it might be long, but at least I would get all the treatment over with at once. Other people might have a shorter operation, but then they needed weeks of radiotherapy or chemotherapy. If you added up all the treatment time, mine was actually shorter. This helped a bit, but I was still anxious.

Finally, I decided that I would look at it like a long flight. I hate long plane journeys, as I can't sleep sitting up. But that has never stopped me booking trips. I just don't think about the flight. I get on the plane, accept that it will be unpleasant and trust that everyone will get me safely to the other side. And that is how I made myself think about the operation.

I spent the weekend in a daze. I didn't want to see anyone. I didn't want to talk about any of it, but there was nothing else I could talk about. I still made sure that I wrote each day.

On the Monday morning, I spoke to a therapist about how I was doing. I had realised that, by nature, I am a worst-case scenario planner. Maybe it is the Emergency Medicine doctor in me. I am always trying to stay at least one step ahead, and I constantly ask myself what is the worst thing that can happen, so that I can prepare for it.

The therapist asked what would be the worst thing that could happen. I said it would either be to die under the anaesthetic or to be in the position where they failed to remove all the cancer.

She said that she understood that it was in my nature to have a worst-case scenario, but did I also have a best-case one? I said yes, that would be that they would get it all out and I would have no stoma. I didn't care what else they had to remove. I didn't care if they gave me a hysterectomy or took out my spleen.

After I spoke to the therapist, I tried to tidy up a little before my sister came the next day. (This information will no doubt shock her, as my flat was still utter chaos when she arrived.) In my bedroom, I found a small bag containing several unwritten postcards. I had bought them a few years earlier for one of our Forum Theatre projects. They were for a lovely exercise that we did at the end. Everyone picked a card and wrote their name on it. The cards were then passed round for everyone else to write a message on it for them. These were the leftover cards that hadn't been picked.

One of them was of a photograph of the top of a grand-looking building but across it, picked out in neon lights, were the words 'Everything Is Going to Be Alright.' As signs go, it was a pretty good one. I started to cry as I held it in my hand, reading and re-reading it. It occurred to me that maybe, just maybe, it could be true. Perhaps I would end up getting my best-case scenario.

I thought back to my previous self, buying it. I wondered what she would have thought of her choice now. For a moment, I imagined that, somewhere inside me, I had known my fate and was sending my future self a message, like a character in a fantastical story. I put the card into my bag and took it to the hospital with me when I went in two days later.

## February 2023: The Promise of Spring

I had to go to a different hospital for my pre-op assessment. I was dreading it. It wasn't just the appointment; it was also having to get there. Combined, the two things overwhelmed me. Then I remembered my conversation with the psychologist. Getting there was another transition. I reassured myself that once I was there, I would feel alright. The hospital wasn't far from my house, but I had never been to it before.

One of the reasons I found it nearly impossible to go out, even to buy bread, was that I just couldn't cope with the process involved. You may not think that there is much process in buying bread but, actually, there is: stand up, decide what to wear, find your shoes, find the shopping bags, decide if you want anything else, find your keys, see if it's raining… The list goes on. Lots of little steps that we normally don't even notice. But all my mental energy was being used to keep the terror of my condition at bay. I struggled to spare any for even the simplest of things.

I ordered my taxi ridiculously early. When the driver asked me when my appointment was, I told him that I had given myself plenty of time.

'No point sitting around being stressed,' I said.

'No,' he replied. 'Stress is not good for you or your baby.'

Here we go again. 'I'm not pregnant,' I answered. 'I have a rare cancer.'

He didn't speak for the rest of the journey. Discomfort radiated from him. Turns out that telling people you have cancer is as much a conversation killer as telling them that you're not pregnant. I wanted to try and make him feel better. But I couldn't think of anything to say.

It was true about me and transitions; once I got to the hospital it was fine. I had my appointment, and everyone was lovely. When I left, it wasn't completely dark. In my old life, this might have been that day when you notice that it is still light as you leave work, the day that reminds you that spring is on its way. I felt a surge of energy and thought about trying to walk some of the way home. I wanted to be outside, I wanted to be in it. But I was exhausted by the time I got to the door, and so I phoned for a taxi.

That night I sat, as usual, on my sofa under my electric blanket. My sister was coming the next day and the day after that I would go into hospital. This would be my last night alone in my flat for... I didn't know how long for, maybe even forever. This was my last normal night.

I ran through the list of everything that I was scared of in my head.

1) I would die under the anaesthetic.

2) I would suffer serious complications under the anaesthetic.

3) I would just not be myself anymore after the anaesthetic.

Listing them like that helped me. I could see that they were unlikely, particularly, the first one. But then came...

4) They wouldn't be able to get it all out and I would have an ileostomy.

I tried to prepare myself for the moment I would find out. But I couldn't. Every time I started, I panicked too much and couldn't finish my thought. Then I thought of the therapist asking me about my best-case scenario. I tried to imagine that, too. It was as if there was a large pair of old-fashioned scales in my head and I needed to balance them. But I couldn't image the best-case scenario either. It was just as painful, but in a different way. It just seemed too good to ever be true. I sat up for a long time. I was reluctant to go to bed, as I wanted to hold on to every last moment of the evening. But in the end, I was too tired and had to admit defeat.

## February 2023: Jelly Belly

My sister arrived. She was to be an absolute superstar over the next few weeks. She was a complete expert now on pseudomyxoma peritonei.

'Are there any positive stories?' I asked.

'Oh, yes,' she said. 'There was one woman who sounded very similar to you. She had the big jelly belly and initially they thought she had ovarian cancer, but then they found out it was PMP. She had the operation you're going to have and was back to normal in six months.'

'Jelly belly?' I asked.

'Yes,' my sister replied. 'That's what they call that big belly you have.'

'Jelly belly,' I said, looking down at my huge abdomen. The biggest irony was that, ever since childhood, I have hated jelly.

The next morning, we got a taxi to the hospital. The driver went up through Kentish Town and Camden. I looked out at the familiar streets. People were walking to work, whilst others were opening their businesses. When we stopped at lights, I watched someone comfort a child who had fallen over and someone else pull on their dachshund's lead as it refused to move.

In my memory, the taxi had tinted windows. But maybe I have imagined that. Everything seemed very quiet. I could see the street, but not really hear it. There was something cinematic about it.

I wondered if this was my last ever view of the world. And if I did see it again, what sort of state would I be in? Would I be the same person; would I still be me? In many ways the idea of not being me, or of being a different me, was harder to get my head around than the idea of being dead.

At the hospital, I was given a wrist band and shown to my room. Sarah and I chatted and then she went to get something to eat. While she was away, the stoma nurse came to visit me. I knew there was a high chance that I would need a stoma. If they didn't get it all out, I would get an ileostomy, which would be at the right side just under my ribs. Even if they did get it out, I might need a colostomy, which would be on my left side, but there was a possibility that it could be reversed later.

She asked if I had any questions. I asked if I could still fly and go on holiday; she said that I could. I asked if I could do Zumba with a stoma; she said that I could. This made me feel slightly happier.

She needed to put stickers on my abdomen for where the stomas should go, if I needed one. When I took off my top, I was shocked by how large my belly — the jelly belly — had become. It was massive. It seemed much bigger than when I went to the GP. My sister came back at this point. She later told me that she, too, was shocked by its size. The stoma nurse asked had I always had an 'outy' belly button. I hadn't, but I did now. I had no idea when that had occurred.

After she left, Sarah and I chatted. I was to be in theatre by 07:00 the next morning, so I told her not to come in to see me before I went. She wanted to, but I said that it was far too early.

Later, she sent me a WhatsApp message asking how I was. I said that I was okay but scared. She replied that I had no need to be scared, that the operation would be fine and, whatever happened, at least I would be a normal size again, and then we could both go home. I found this incredibly reassuring, and it made me smile. It still does, whenever I think of it.

I sat and waited for the next day to come. I phoned my mum and we both cried. I felt incredibly guilty about what I was putting her through. A few friends texted to say that they were thinking of me. And I prayed. I had been a sporadic pray-er in adulthood, but had taken it up in earnest since this had all started. I thanked God for sparing me ovarian cancer and asked could they now please get all the pseudomyxoma out.

I remembered a story that was often told in my family. Back when my mum was at school, she was going to do her Home Economics exam. The way the exam worked was that everyone was allocated, at random, three items to cook — a starter, a main course and dessert — from a selection of set dishes on the syllabus. They had been practising for weeks.

Now, my mum was the star of the Home Economics class and could cook everything except for one thing: the Swiss Roll. No matter what she did, her Swiss Roll always cracked. As she was leaving for the exam, my grandmother called after her, 'I'll say a wee prayer for you.'

'Yes,' replied my mother. 'Pray I don't get the Swiss Roll.'

My grandmother was a very devout woman and understood a thing or two about prayer.

'No,' she replied. 'I'll pray that whatever you get, God will help you deal with it.'

My mother claims that part of her wasn't surprised when the exam started, and she drew the Swiss Roll. There was a certain inevitability about it. When the time came, she removed it from the oven with a heavy heart. But when she unwrapped it, there it was, absolutely perfect, not a crack in sight. Apparently, the examiner said, 'You must tell me your secret. I can never get mine to work.'

Or maybe she didn't; maybe, over time, I just added that bit in myself. Maybe I added in lots of the details. But that's the thing about a really good story: there comes a point where you can no longer tell where it ends, and you begin.

I thought about my grandmother for a few moments. And then I prayed that whatever was to happen to me, God would help me to deal with it.

It almost felt like the night before you go on holiday and, irrationally, I fretted that I would somehow sleep in and miss my operation. I was awake in plenty of time, though, and up and showered and ready to go.

The anaesthetist came in to have a quick chat, and then my surgeon. It was the first time I had met him face-to-face. He explained again what he was going to do. As he left, I surprised myself by feeling the urge to try and make a joke.

'I hope you've had a good breakfast,' I said.

He smiled. 'Remember, we do this regularly.'

I found this immensely reassuring. I recalled a work colleague who was an excellent doctor, a cardiologist, once remarking that he often said to patients, 'I know this is a huge day for you, but remember, for me it's just a day doing my job.'

Shortly afterwards, a health care assistant came and walked me down to the operating theatre. She chatted away to me as we walked along the corridor. I felt huge in the lift, like I was taking up far too much room. I remembered my sister's text from the day before. Hopefully, whatever else happened, at least some of the jelly belly would be gone by the time I woke up. If I woke up, that is.

I went into the anaesthetic room and climbed up onto the trolley. The nurse went to help me, but I felt it was important that I tried to do it by myself. She talked to me as the anaesthetist put in an intravenous cannula. When I looked, I was surprised to see that it was a brown one, the largest size. I remembered point number three on my list of things that I would focus on: 'I have good, big veins.'

Then the nurse took my hand and started chatting to me. For the briefest of moments, I thought I saw her exchange a look with the anaesthetist.

# February 2023: Magic

I was trying to concentrate, and I couldn't. It was very important that I concentrated because if I didn't, I would lose it; I could feel it slipping away from me and I was scrambling to hold onto it, to ignore the voices.

'Heidi, Heidi.'

I realised that I was dreaming but, in that moment, the dreaming world was as real and as important as the waking world and I wasn't ready to be pulled out of it just yet.

'Wake up, Heidi, time to wake up.'

Too late. The last remnants of the dream slipped away.

For a long time, I tried to think of the best way to describe how it felt to wake up after my operation, but I couldn't. I couldn't quite believe it. How could the operation be over? This thing that I had dreaded: how could it be over? I hadn't even realised that it had begun and already it was finished. It was fantastical, like magic, and so, in the end, I realised that that was the best way to describe it. It felt magical. I would never again make jokes about anaesthetists merely putting people to sleep and waking them up again. Now, they were just one step away from being wizards.

Several people have asked if being a doctor made my whole experience better or worse. The answer is both. My insights made some things more scary, other things less. Waking up in ITU was definitely one of the times when it helped. The environment was close enough to the resus room in the Emergency Department to be familiar to me; there was nothing alien or frightening about it, whereas, for my sister when she visited, it was alarming. Every time a machine beeped, she would feel anxious, whereas I knew that it was just that my antibiotics had run through.

When I woke up, I looked at the clock. It was just after eight o'clock.

'Is it morning or night?' I asked.

'Morning,' was the reply. Friday morning. They had kept me sedated and intubated overnight. I felt no pain whatsoever, but I was aware that I had a lot of tubes coming out of me. I lay back and let myself feel relieved.

I could read the sounds of the ITU like a tracker reads the noises of the forest. I knew from the way people were talking — the speed, volume and pitch of their voices and something else too, the atmosphere in the room — that no-one was worried about me. That meant that I was stable; I was a routine post-op patient.

I couldn't believe it. I had achieved the first three things on my list. I hadn't died under anaesthetic; I hadn't had any major complications; and I felt entirely myself. My train of thought felt continuous from the time I was in the anaesthetic room. There was a slight blip caused by the operation and then it had picked up exactly from where it had left off. I was so happy and relieved.

But I was also aware that points one to three were the easy wins. There was still the big one, point number four: had they managed to get everything out?

I had partly rehearsed this moment in my mind, although this was one of the thoughts that I had struggled to complete. Also, when I had tried to prepare for it, I didn't know what sort of state I was going to be in when I woke up in ITU. But, as far as I could tell, I was pretty normal. I could move all four of my limbs and, mentally, I just felt like me.

I knew that, if they had been unable to get it all out, I would have an ileostomy, so all I had to do was feel for one on my right side. I was reluctant to do this. I was just so happy that I hadn't died, I didn't want to spoil it. I just wanted to enjoy being happy for a while.

But I realised that this was more of my usual 'it's not the waiting it's the finding out' attitude. And, let's be honest, that hadn't worked out too well for me so far. I remembered what the psychologist had said. Once I got somewhere, I seemed to be fine; the problem was the transition. And finding out was just a type of transition.

If they hadn't got it all out, then I might as well start dealing with it. I said a little prayer, and slid my hands beneath the sheets and under my gown. A large dressing ran the entire length of my abdomen. My fingers brushed against something that felt like plastic. But it was too low for where an ileostomy would be. It felt like a plastic tube, and I realised that it must be some kind of surgical drain.

I felt up to under my ribs but I couldn't feel anything. Surely, I couldn't have got away with it, dodged another bullet? I felt on the left side to see if I had a colostomy, but I could not feel anything there either. I just lay there. I was too scared to believe that they had got everything out. What if I was wrong? Maybe I should check again.

In some ways, it was harder the second time, but I forced myself. I poked around my abdomen more firmly this time, but I still couldn't locate anything that felt like either an ileostomy or a colostomy. Maybe it was under the big dressing. But why would they cover a stoma with a dressing?

I was just about to feel for a third time when I saw someone waving to me from the door. She looked excited.

'You didn't get a stoma, you didn't get a stoma — they got it all out.'

It took me a few seconds to recognise that it was the stoma nurse from yesterday. She came into the room.

'I know,' I said. 'I know.'

I don't remember who took the other one's hand, but suddenly we were holding hands. I was crying and, in my memory, so was she.

'I'm just so happy,' I sobbed.

And I was. It was the happiest I have ever been. I had never felt that happy before and I don't know if I ever will again. To be honest, I'm relieved about that. Even now, when I think about it, I just start to cry. That kind of happiness was just too much to bear. It was too intense. I felt like a character in a story who has been touched by the hand of God. It was a kind of wildness that no human being can sustain for long. I lay there, feeling euphoric. I couldn't understand how or why I had been so lucky. I had got my best possible outcome. I must be the luckiest person alive.

After a while, the physio came in. She explained that they would try to get me walking as soon as possible, but that day she only wanted to see what I was like sitting up. She and the nurse helped me roll onto my side. The plan was that she would count to three and then lift me.

When she got to three, I instinctively tried to sit up myself. She told me that I had done most of the work. This was apparently rare on the first day after the operation.

'It's all the Zumba,' I said. 'I do a lot of Zumba classes. I have this instructor called Onyeka; she's really fantastic. The fact that I can sit up is a testament to her.'

I felt it was really important to talk about Zumba. At that point, I saw my sister standing at the door, watching. Sarah later told me that she was stunned. She had expected me to be lying down, and out of it for at least three days. She couldn't believe that I was sitting up, chatting and lucid.

I made her tell me exactly what she had done the day before, the day of my operation. For a while, I was fascinated by that day, as I felt that I had not really lived it. It was a length of time I had not experienced. Over the next few weeks, I found out that lots of people had thought about me or prayed for me during those hours.

People of all different faiths prayed for me: Jewish, Islam, Christian and Hindu. Alison, my best friend at home, told me that she couldn't settle all day. When she came back from work, she took down all her lampshades and washed them. She also shouted my name out every hour. She couldn't explain why. She just thought I might, on some level, know that she was calling out to me, and it would help bring me back safely. I can never think or write about any of this without crying.

## February 2023: Teeny Tiny

That night, I had horrible nightmares. I was walking through a large house. Each room contained a different nightmare. I woke up a few times, sweating and shaking. At some point, in that strange state between awake and asleep, I understood that this, somehow, was the terror: all the fear beneath the denial I had constructed over the last year in order not to deal with what was going on. I had the sense that I was now dismantling it and I should just persevere with the nightmares, as they were part of what I needed to do to heal. The next morning when I woke, I felt mentally better. I had been scared for a very long time, but now I felt less so.

I stayed on ITU for a week. I didn't mind it. In all honesty, I much preferred being a patient on ITU to being a doctor there. All Emergency Medicine doctors have to spend time on ITU as part of their training. I hated it. I was an atrocious ITU doctor; it played to all of my weaknesses and none of my strengths.

All my career, I have had a good relationship with my colleagues and the utmost respect for them. But I loved the nurses that looked after me in ITU and later on the ward. It was a different kind of relationship. They were the people who were with me when I was at my most scared and vulnerable.

On Friday night, the first night I was awake on the unit, the nurse who had been looking after me when I was admitted, came to say hello.

'I cared for you last night,' she said.

I thought a lot about that phrase over the next few months. I have said it to people and have heard others use it. I suppose I have always thought of it the medical sense, cared for as in provided medical treatment. But I realised that, when I was suspended between worlds, alone and powerless, she had been with me and had cared for me in all senses of the phrase.

The ITU consultant who had admitted me also came in. He told me that he had given me twelve litres of fluid. This is a huge amount. I required so much because, as well as having a big operation, my body was adjusting to losing so much fluid in the form of all the ascites. Also, the chemotherapy that was put inside me was heated to a high temperature.

The physio came each day to get me walking. I was scared, and had to force myself. I was hindered by seven surgical drains: five in my abdomen and two chest drains. I also had other intravenous lines, for pain relief, medications and nutrition. I would use my drip stand for support whilst the physio walked beside me. One of the nurses had to walk behind carrying all my drains. I imagined us as a kind of surreal procession.

Even that short walk exhausted me. The nurses deserve a lot of credit because they acted as such cheerleaders in getting me moving. Every day, I walked a little further.

On one of my last nights on the unit, it transpired that the nurse looking after me was originally from the same part of Ireland as me. We chatted about home, and about my operation. I mentioned the twelve litres of fluid.

'Gosh,' he said, 'and you're such a tiny, petite, little thing.'

What the hell? I hadn't seen myself since the operation, but at no time in my life had anyone ever described me as a tiny, petite, little thing.

Toto, I have the feeling that we're not in Kansas, anymore.

My drains were removed in stages and, finally, on the Friday, the last of them came out. Now I could be transferred to the ward. Despite, originally, being scared of the idea of having to go to ITU, I was now scared at the thought of leaving it. I felt safe there; it had been my whole world for the last few days — such intense days; they seemed like a lifetime.

I was moved that evening. It wasn't the same room as before, but it was the same view. The last time I had seen it, I hadn't known what was going to happen to me and I felt that same joyous wonder that it had all worked out.

As I went to sleep, I reflected on my year so far. The Friday before I had woken up in ITU; the one before that was when I had freaked out as I was told that I would be going into hospital the next week. Two Fridays before that, I thought I had ovarian cancer and was going to die; the Friday before that was when I had seen my GP and the one before that was when I had made myself make the appointment. A week and a day before that was when my mum had told me I needed to see a doctor.

I struggled to get my head around it all. I felt as if I had lived years of my life when nothing much had really happened; when, certainly, nothing much seemed to have changed. So far, 2023 was shaping up to be some year.

I still had two intravenous lines. One of these was attached to my patient-controlled analgesia, and the other was to give me intravenous feeding. These were both taken down on the Monday evening and I was finally free.

Whilst I was in ITU, the nurses had washed me. When I was moved to the ward, I had been able to wash myself with wet wipes. But now I was able to go into the bathroom. Finally, I got a good look at myself. I took off my gown and stared at my naked reflection. I couldn't quite take it in. I was tiny. Not slender or slim or skinny: I was teeny tiny. I looked at myself from all angles. I couldn't believe that my body was capable of being that small.

I was as unnerved by tiny me as I had been by enormous me. This new body was as alien as the jelly belly one had been. All my curves had disappeared. I had no idea how to be this shape either.

There was something scary about my new body. Despite being undeniably thin, it wasn't that attractive. Huge folds of flesh hung off me, from my abdomen but also my legs. I was like a deflated balloon. There was something shrunken and wizened about my appearance. I could see quite how emaciated my limbs had become. They were like sticks. I had obvious muscle-wasting. It was like being in a fairy tale or *Alice in Wonderland*. One minute, I was enormous — and then I had gone to sleep and woken up tiny. For all of that last year, I hadn't been putting on weight; it wasn't the menopause; I hadn't not tried hard enough; and I hadn't failed. I had just been very, very sick.

I looked at my reflection for a long time, trying to come to terms with it. Approximately twenty minutes later, I was buying myself new clothes online. I had absolutely no idea what size I was nor how long I would remain that way. I felt a familiar stab of guilt about buying clothes that I didn't really need. But, I told myself, apart from the very large tee shirts, I hadn't really bought myself anything the previous year. Also — surely, I deserved a treat?

Now that I was free of all my attachments — or accessories, as I had taken to calling them — it was much easier to walk. I had come on well and the physio no longer needed to see me. She suggested that I should walk round the ward a few times each day. The first time, I got my sister to accompany me. I was hesitant, but soon relaxed. Sarah had hurt her back that morning so, at one point, she had to tell me to slow down.

The next day, I told myself that I should be a big, brave girl and just get on and do it. Then I had an idea. I put my headphones on, and found some tracks from the Zumba classes on YouTube. As soon as I heard that music, I felt a little rush and started to smile. Joni Mitchell sings about the kind of loss that you only notice after something has gone. But there is another kind of loss, that is so painful that you can only deal with it by blocking it out. This is what I had done with my Zumba classes.

But, slowly doing laps of the ward, I realised that maybe one day I could go back. Listening to the music, I was back in the gym. I could see Onyeka at the front, and lots of the other women who were regulars, some whose names I knew, others whose I didn't. I could feel the sheer joy in the room. I was just so happy, I started to cry and had to wipe the tears away before anyone noticed and one of the nurses came to check if I was alright.

Round and round I walked, the Zumba songs playing like a soundtrack. On the outside, I was somewhere that felt reassuringly familiar. It was comforting watching the nurses getting on with their jobs or laughing at the desk. Inside my head, I was dancing.

## February 2023: Looking-Glass World

I made good progress. Initially, they said I might need to stay in for around three weeks, but I was discharged after two weeks and two days.

My surgeon came to see me before I left. He told me that, for a while, he had thought that he might not be able to get it all off my small bowel, but he had persevered and done it. Now I had to go home and focus on healing.

I thanked him for everything that he had done. He did something that I have seen doctors do numerous times, and may even have done myself. He tried to brush off my thanks by saying, 'I was just doing my job.'

I shook my head. 'No,' I said. I may even have said, 'I'm not taking that,' or maybe I just thought it. But I felt very strongly that I wasn't taking it. He may have just been doing his job, but he had done it very well. His job had made a whole world of difference to me. He may just have been doing his job, but what a job that was. What a job we all do, I thought.

On the morning of my discharge, the nurse specialist took down my huge dressing and I saw my scar for the first time. It ran the whole length of my abdomen. They had also removed my belly button, as the tumour can metastasise there. Painstakingly, she took out all the tiny staples.

Then it was time to go, and I said goodbye to all the nurses and got into the lift. The last time I had been in it, I had felt very big. Now I felt very small. I waited in reception whilst Sarah called for a taxi. It struck me that she was so much more familiar with this part of the hospital than me.

We walked out into the sunshine. Time had moved on in the outside world. That's what time does, it's always moving on; it's just that, usually, we don't notice, as we're too busy with other things. It was now late February, and I could feel that the arrival of spring was definitely in the air.

I looked out of the taxi window. It was the reverse of the journey that I had made just over two weeks ago, wondering if it would be my last. Or my last as the person that I was. And yet here I was, just myself — a tiny version of myself — going home. Everything had worked out alright. I still couldn't quite believe it.

I watched the familiar streets of Camden and Kentish Town go by. To me, they had a shiny, sparkling quality — the joy of a normal day, a normal life, and I was still part of it.

My mother and sister had been concerned as to how I was going to manage the stairs up to my flat. Sarah had counted that I would have to walk up fifty-seven steps. But she had come up with a plan. She had bought a camping seat. I could take a break on each of the landings.

'I can even bring you a cup of tea or coffee, if you want,' she said. 'There is no rush.'

As she unlocked the front door, I took a deep breath and walked up all the stairs without stopping. It was easier than it had been after doing a shift at work, then walking home with my shopping, not to mention carrying the jelly belly. The nurse specialists had told me that, sometimes, people who have soldiered on with their symptoms find it easier post-op because, no matter how difficult it is, it is an improvement on what it had been before.

The next big surprise was my flat. Whilst I had been in hospital, my sister had cleaned it and had all the broken things fixed. I couldn't believe it. My flat will never be immaculate, but it had become homely and cosy. I remembered, before Christmas, thinking that everything was beyond repair, yet here we all were, mended.

As I made my way to the sofa, I caught a glimpse of my teeny tiny reflection in the mirror: the mirror where I had, once upon a time, scrutinised the jelly belly. I felt I had well and truly slipped through the looking-glass and come home to a parallel world.

The next few weeks had a dreamlike quality. I was now a tiny, little person living in my tidy, little flat. My sister fussed round me constantly. When we went out, she often had to open heavy doors for me, as I was too frail to do it myself. For the first time in my life, I had no appetite, though I needed to eat. Digestion frequently gave me severe stomach cramps. I was constantly trying to force myself to eat small amounts, rather than diet.

Several of my friends had visited me in the hospital. And now people climbed all the stairs to my flat to see me. They looked at me in what seemed like a combination of amazement and awe. They were amazed by how well I looked, and in awe that I was so positive after such an operation.

I pointed out that I looked well because I was no longer trying to carry round litres of ascites whilst anaemic and malnourished. And I was positive, as I felt that the nightmare was over: not just the trauma of the last few weeks, but the ordeal of the previous year.

Everyone wanted to care for me. People cooked and baked and came to fuss round me, giving my sister a break. I don't think I have ever felt quite so loved in all my life.

I was contacted by the nurse specialist from the hospital to check how I was doing. She told me that the cytology had come back, and I had had a low-grade tumour (gentle dog as opposed to angry one). I would be under surveillance for twenty years, which would involve yearly CT scans. I asked if it would come back. Again, I knew the answer, which is that nobody knows, but things were as positive as they could be. I asked her to thank my surgeon, and everyone involved in my care.

'I will never not be grateful,' I said.

Afterwards, I thought about that line and wondered if it were true. Would I stop being grateful one day? If I was lucky enough to lead a long life after this, would all the tiny annoyances and irritations, all the disappointments and heartaches, eventually rise up and choke this feeling? In the end, I decided maybe, but what I needed to do was keep the idea of gratitude always in my head, as an aspiration rather than a promise.

One day, I went into work. I needed to get the stitches removed from my drain sites and I also had to get a blood test. I could have gone to my GP, but I wanted to go and see everyone. I also wanted them to see me; to see that I had survived, and also to see that I wasn't pregnant but was, in fact, now teeny tiny.

Whilst there, I saw my CT scan. It was terrifying: the sort of thing that belonged in a textbook for everyone to gaze at in horrified fascination. The doctor in me still couldn't quite get her head around the fact that she had been that patient. My whole abdominal cavity was full of fluid, full to bursting. The report described it as a massive, tense ascites. It had squashed up all my internal organs. My liver and kidneys were tiny, and my gastro-intestinal tract was squashed into a corner. I imagine if I had left things for much longer, I would have developed a bowel obstruction. I couldn't believe that I had been working right up until a week before the ascites was aspirated.

Then I looked round the Emergency Department, with all the patients on trolleys squashed into every available bit of space. It was as if my body had been a metaphor for the department and the department had been a metaphor for my body. And I was so relieved not to have to be dealing with either of them.

## March 2023: Home

After a few weeks, Sarah and I flew back home to Ireland. We planned the trip scrupulously. Sarah said she was looking forward to a Bacardi and Coke on the plane as she would finally feel that she could relax. That was when it struck me properly how stressful she had found the whole thing. She had never shown it and had looked after me so well.

We watched the progression of the drinks trolley. Just before it reached us, the crew stopped and pushed it to the back of the plane. Then they rushed down to the front. We looked at each other. A few seconds later, the call came: 'If there is doctor or nurse or anyone with medical or first aid training, could they please make themselves known to the cabin crew.'

I shook my head. The call came again.

'I can't,' I said.

On the third call, I had to accept that no-one else was volunteering. I got up shakily and made my way down the plane, with Sarah behind me.

'Hi,' I said. 'I'm a doctor, an Emergency Medicine consultant.'

The cabin crew let out great sighs of relief.

'I'm going to have to sit down, though,' I added.

I introduced myself to the patient. It felt strange to be doing this again. I could feel my brain creaking back into life. I hadn't been away that long, but already I felt rusty.

A family friend collected us from the airport. He wanted to get the car and bring it right outside, but I wanted to walk the short distance to the carpark. I just wanted to prove to myself that I could do it.

We drove the sixty miles home to Portrush. It is a journey that I am very familiar with, having done it regularly for the past thirty-five years, ever since I left to go to university. It seemed to be both very normal and remarkable at the same time. There is a part of the journey where you turn onto the coast road and suddenly see Portrush and the sea. It looked dazzling in the evening light, and I started to cry, but turned so that no-one could see. When I arrived home, my mother looked at me in amazement. I'm not sure if it was because I had come through so much, or because I was so teeny tiny, or a combination of both.

For the first few weeks, I stayed with Sarah. We drove up to her apartment. It was a crisp, clear night with a sky full of stars. Living in London: you never see the stars. For a time, I completely forgot that they even existed and then, one day, with a shock, I remembered all about them and wondered where they had gone. The answer was, obviously, nowhere; they were just hidden.

I was very frail and in pain a lot of the time. I still got severe stomach cramps whenever I ate. The first meal of the day was particularly difficult. I didn't care, though. I was just so happy that I no longer had the jelly belly and that I had survived.

I quickly got into a new routine. When I arrived, it was mid-March, and mostly wet and windy. My instructions were to walk every day, but it was easy to use the weather as an excuse not to leave the house. However, after about a fortnight, it brightened up and Sarah and I went out one Saturday. I enjoyed the fresh air, but felt shaky on my skinny legs: like Bambi learning to walk. It wasn't just the weather that was making me reluctant; I was also scared of leaving my sister. She had been with me every day since the operation, and I felt anxious at the thought of not having her close by. When I realised that, I knew that I had to go out on my own.

The following Monday, I waited until my breakfast stomach cramps had settled and then set out. Portrush is a peninsula, and on each side is a beach. I walked down to the West Strand, the shorter of the two beaches.

It took me about twenty minutes to get there. There was a huge ship in the bay. I sat and watched it for a while, and then walked back.

The next day, I walked a little further, and the day after that, further still. In time, I was able to walk along the whole of the West Strand and then the longer East Strand too. That became the thing that I did: I walked.

At the end of March, Alison came and took me out for a drive. We drove east along the coast road. The day was like a cliché of spring. If it had been a painting, it would have been a Victorian watercolour — the sort of thing used to decorate biscuit tins or tea caddies and dismissed as twee. The sea sparkled to the left of us, and to the right the fields rolled. What's more, they were full of lambs gambolling and there were great tubs of daffodils outside all the houses. The day felt as if it had been freshly washed and hung out to dry in the light March wind.

We drove down to a small village by the sea and walked along the beach. Alison took a selfie of the two of us. It was a tradition we had started over twenty years before on holiday and for the last decade, it had been the first thing that we had done every New Year's Eve. But, of course, this year we had missed it. This was our New Year selfie, only three months late.

Later, when I looked at it, that is what struck me the most: that it was only three months late. The last time I had seen Alison was the night I could hardly walk from the car to the restaurant; the night my mother told me that I needed to see a doctor.

Then, it had seemed impossible that I would ever be in a better place. Even with my wild imagination, I couldn't conceive of such a thing. And yet here I was, in a day that was so perfect that it almost didn't seem real. In only three months, I had somehow managed to negotiate all that shame and fear and horribleness, and now I was standing on a beach in the sunshine, laughing. It felt as if I had made an archetypal journey, through the darkness of winter and out into the brightness of spring.

## April 2023: The Beach

My surgeon had told me that I had to go home and concentrate on healing. So that was the question. How do you heal yourself or let yourself heal?

I was surprised when I realised that I, a doctor, knew very little about healing. I knew lots about diagnosing conditions and sometimes not even diagnosing them but stratifying risk; I knew how to decide when it was safe to send someone home or if they needed to come into hospital; I knew about treatment — mostly the immediate management of things — and a little about long-term care. But I really knew nothing of healing.

I started to walk along the beach each day. That walk and the beach became two of the most important things in the new world in which I was now living. There was something important about walking the same walk every day. I imagined people asking: didn't you get bored of it? But how I felt about it wasn't the point. It wasn't about excitement or stimulation or novelty. It was about healing. There was a safety in it being the same every day. I had had all the excitement that I needed for quite some time. I had had enough new experiences.

And, down on the beach, things never stayed the same. Very quickly, I saw that every day was different. The beach changed in so many ways, not least whether the tide was in or out. When the tide was high, even the hard sand by the water's edge was softer. I learned that the tide was always further in than it looked.

The atmosphere felt different, too. When the tide was out, things were mellow, reflective. The beach exposed its wrinkled underbelly. A vast expanse of polished sand was left behind, containing multiple deltas and lagoons that would reflect the sky back up at me, so that some days it felt as if I was walking amongst the clouds.

When the tide was high, things were much more energetic. Sometimes, the sea was frisky, playful like a puppy, and would chase me right up the beach. Other days, it was wilder still. It gave the air a rawness that made my eyes water and scraped at my skin.

I began to recognise the people walking their dogs: the lady with the greyhound in the purple raincoat; the man with the spaniel who always had a big stick. They would smile and say hello.

I could have spent all day there. I would stand and watch where the waves first broke, surprisingly far out at sea, and follow them until they came into the shore. I loved watching the way the gulls took off sideways into the wind. There weren't only gulls down on the beach; there was a surprising number of crows, who, even more surprisingly, frequently hung out with the gulls. Were they friends? I always felt that they were up to no good. They just had that air about them. I would think up all sorts of scenarios for them.

I couldn't help but laugh at myself when it hit me that this was what I did, now that my main 'job' was to walk the beach: I thought up stories about seagulls and crows. But was that any more a waste of my time and mental energy than trying to explain, yet again, why we were failing to meet government performance targets in an overcrowded, understaffed, exhausted and demoralised department?

I began to notice things: flowers that would appear some mornings and be gone the next; pieces of driftwood; jellyfish. I was also more aware of how I felt each day, of how some days I had more energy than others. I began to notice how I felt emotionally too; what sort of mood I was in.

But none of it mattered down on the beach. I didn't have to feel any particular way. I didn't need to take my A-game to the beach. I just went as I was, and by the time I came home I would be different. Each day, the beach changed me slightly.

I noticed my thoughts — how they would float across my consciousness before they disappeared like the shadows of gulls that sometimes flitted across me as I walked. The beach became my whole world, a world of sea, sky, water and sand.

Previously, everything in my life was overcrowded, both within the department and inside my body. But out here, it was all wide-open spaces. My life, which had previously felt so contracted, began to feel expansive again. I felt space open up inside my head too, and I was able to think about everything that had happened to me over the last year.

How had I managed to walk around for as long as I did with the jelly belly? I began to get a glimpse into the vastness of the shame and fear that I had also been carrying around with me. As time went on, I was to discover, from various conversations with friends, that they were horrified too; horrified that they had not noticed or, if they had, had pushed it to some far corner of their mind. Their relationship with the whole thing was as complex as mine. Many of them expressed guilt that they hadn't said anything. They had nothing to feel guilty about. For most of the time, they had thought that I was putting on weight too.

Perhaps one of the most fascinating insights came from a conversation with a person who asked, if I could go back in time, what would I have liked people to have said? And, sitting there, I could easily recall the deep shame that I had felt. Despite everything, I still wouldn't have wanted anyone to say anything. I had actively repelled people. So, on some level, I think that I stopped people from saying anything.

But it did make me wonder why we, as a society, have so demonised putting on weight that I ended up like this? How did weight and shape become something that I felt such a deep sense of shame about?

I was amazed at how I had been able to deny what was going on with me for so long. Looking back, I could see all the times my subconscious had been screaming at me that something was wrong, and I chose to ignore it.

My subconscious had been spot on. I thought about the day that I had seen my reflection and the PG Wodehouse comment about the tubby little chap who had been poured into his clothes and hadn't said "when!" had come into my head. That was the most precise description of what was happening to me. I thought about the story I had written about the robin who was getting bigger and bigger as it bloated up with badness.

Part of me was appalled that I had dragged myself into work in the condition that I was in. But the part of me that had trained back in the 1990s felt pride that I had kept going. Then I was appalled at myself for thinking that. It was nothing to be proud of.

But that's the culture of the NHS; it encourages us to keep going because, the truth is, that's what it relies on. Doing something for nothing is seen as a virtue and, on occasions, as proof of your dedication. There's nothing wrong with occasionally going the extra mile for your patients or your colleagues; we all do. But there is something seriously wrong with the system when it would fall apart if we didn't.

I spoke to a therapist about it. I said I felt that, at some point, I had completely dissociated from my own body. She agreed that I probably had. It's a common response to trauma and I was obviously traumatised by what I was going through: my illness, but also my intolerable working conditions.

Working in that environment of constant crisis had made it harder for me to recognise, accept and deal with the fact that my body was also in crisis. It also made it much easier to hide what was going on, from myself, and my colleagues. They too were having to deal with so much chaos, just surviving from one day to the next. They didn't have the bandwidth to clock what was going on with me. I later learned that it was only in December that they had reached a point where they noticed and began to voice concerns. Then Lucy had spoken to me. Our team structure had been so fragmented by everything that it had been easy for me to fall through the cracks.

I often think back to that conversation with the other doctors on my team, when we discussed the rarest condition that we had ever seen in an emergency department. I could appreciate the irony that it was actually me. There I was, hiding in plain sight, with my pseudomyxoma peritonei.

I genuinely laugh every time I think of this. And, in time, I imagined that I could hear someone else laughing in the background: the ghost of the MRCP Part 1 exam, having the final word. Who knew that it would turn out to have had such a sense of humour?

I sometimes wondered when it had all started. I thought back to February 2020, just before I went to Morocco, when I had the bad stomach pains. Was it then? I remembered that, at that time, I had occasionally had the sense that something was terribly wrong with me. But then COVID came, and the world went into meltdown, and I forgot all about it.

I got up each morning at 06:30 to write, just as I had done every day since the start of the pandemic. I finished the story about the robin being bloated up with badness. I could now see that it was another way my subconscious must have been screaming at me about what was happening to my body. I had written it right up until the day before I went into hospital, and I felt that I owed it to the story to finish it.

Then I began to write about the jelly belly and the previous year; about what had happened to my body and also how hard it had been to work in the NHS over the last few years. I wrote to try and make some sense of it all. I don't know if I did; if I ever will. But by writing my story, I owned it, and it didn't — and still doesn't — own me.

When I walked along the beach, I also thought about a lot of other stuff: a lifetime's worth of it. Disappointments, regrets, failed relationships, and other things that did not work out in the way that I had wanted. Some of this made it into my writing; much more of it didn't. It would float into my head for a while until I let go of it, and then it would float away again. I began to think of it like the things that the sea washed up on the shore each day. Every morning, as I walked down to the beach, I would wonder what the tide would have brought in for me.

So, when I was told to go home and heal, my first question was how? — and my second one was exactly how far back do I need to go?

## May 2023: The Dolphin

One day, in early May, I was walking along the beach. The weather was more like March, bright and blustery. The sea chased me up the beach.

A mother called out, 'Run, Harry, run.'

I turned to see a small boy with his arms outstretched like wings and his coat loose around his shoulders and fastened at his neck to make it look like a cape. He was running up the beach, screaming with laughter.

'Faster,' called his mother. 'Faster.'

And suddenly I wanted to run too. I wanted to make my coat like a cape and stretch my arms out like angel wings. And I wanted to run, run along the beach. Of course, I didn't, but I could feel the wind behind me, egging me on. Out on the sea, it lifted up a kite surfer and he flew along beside me.

I started to walk faster. I was amazed at my speed. I was so aware of the way my feet felt as they made contact with the ground. My heel hit it first and then my foot tilted forward onto the ball which bounced it up again. I could feel the movement pass up through my legs: how my muscles tightened, first my hamstrings, then my thighs and then my bottom.

Faster and faster, I walked, propelled by the wind. I took deep breaths and felt my lungs expand, as if for the first time, with the sea air. It was exhilarating. And I forgot about everything. I forgot about the jelly belly and the operation, the previous year and why I was there down on the beach. I only realised that I had forgotten when I remembered again with a jolt.

Then it hit me: I felt like me. My surgeon had said that, around three months after the operation, some people suddenly realise that they feel like themselves again. He was spot on; it was two months and three weeks.

It was wondrous there on the beach, with the sun and the sea and the wind. But I couldn't help thinking that, most wondrous of all, was me. I had been gifted that rarest of things, something that I had believed was the preserve of fairy tales and bible stories: I had been gifted a miracle.

I thought of myself as a small child, sitting cross-legged on a dusty floor, listening to stories of such things, and wondered what I would have thought if I had been told then that I would grow up to get my very own miracle.

And why on earth, in this world that sometimes seems so full of incalculable pain and suffering, had I, out of so many people, been given one? I thought of all the patients that I had seen die, and those I had met whilst they were dying, and of a surprisingly high number of doctors who died whilst still working. Why me? Why had I been lucky? In amongst the gratitude, I felt a tiny flash of guilt. I started to cry, and put on my sunglasses.

There was a Zumba class on Friday nights. I checked with the nurse specialist from Basingstoke, and she told me that I could go, but to take things easy to begin with. I felt both anxious and excited. As soon as the music started, though, I was able to dance, and I could hardly believe it; it was as if I had never stopped. I cried with joy as I walked home.

In July, Lucy came to visit me. As we sat eating fish and chips by the sea, I remembered that Friday back at the end of January when I thought that I had ovarian cancer, and she came and had coffee with me. I had said that if I got through things, we would treat ourselves to a few days by the sea. Neither of us had believed it; we both thought that I was going to die. Yet here we were, just as we said we would be. It scarcely seemed possible.

As I got stronger, I knew that it was bringing me closer to the time when I would be able to return to my old life and I was shocked to find that part of me felt sad about this. I had grown to love spending my days on the beach with nothing to think about other than getting better. I felt anxious about returning to the normal world and the chaos of work. Even harder to admit was that I had begun to enjoy being frail and constantly cared for. I did not feel under any pressure to hide my vulnerability. There was a grief in getting well again. But I understood that I had to let go of all those feelings. I tried not to think about leaving, and just enjoyed each day that I had.

My old shape started to return. My curves came back, and my skinny legs grew bigger and more muscular. I knew I looked healthier, but part of me couldn't let go of the idea that I had looked so much better when I was skinnier. I was just too conditioned to stop believing that the smaller you are, the better you look. Even after everything I'd been through, I still couldn't let go of that idea. I had to keep reminding myself that partly I had been so small because I had muscle-wasting. I was angry with myself for not being able to stop this way of thinking and embrace my natural shape.

I never had a moment when I decided that I would go back to work. Rather, at some point, it changed in my head from 'if' to 'when'. I had been told to take at least six months off. My sick note was to the end of August. By July, I was walking up to ten miles every day on the beach. It made sense to plan to go back at the start of September. I had felt negative about work for a long time — but, for a long time before that, I had loved it. Once, before things had gone crazy, it had sustained me through some bad times. I wanted to go back to work in good health, to see how I really felt about it.

I was sad to leave home and my family, though. And I was sad to leave the beach. By walking the same walk along it every day, it was as if I had become part of the landscape. I had travelled with it through spring into summer and I wanted to continue into the autumn and winter.

On one of my last days, I spent time saying goodbye to both beaches. I wrote 'thank you' in the sand with a piece of driftwood. Medicine and the NHS had diagnosed and treated me. They had undoubtedly saved me, but it was the beach that had healed me. Again, I would always be grateful.

The following day, I saw a dolphin playing in the waves. I imagined it to be the spirit of the bay. When I told a friend, she asked if I felt that it had come to say goodbye to me. Actually, I didn't. I felt that the dolphin was absorbed in what it was doing and was unaware of my presence. But I did feel that I had caught a glimpse of something of the deep; something that you rarely get to see. I felt privileged.

## Returning: September 2023

At the end of August, I went back to work. I walked up to the hospital on my first day. Walking was one of the things that had helped heal me and I was determined to keep it going. It may not have been the beach, but there were still things to look at, and it was good to be outside.

As I approached the Emergency Department entrance, I remembered the day that I went for my colonoscopy and thought that I would never use this entrance again. The department was completely unchanged. It was still overcrowded, and everyone was incredibly stressed. People were still trying to do their best in an impossible situation.

Touchingly, they were all delighted to see me again. Everyone told me how well I looked. Some people, who have known me for a long time, said it was the best that they had ever seen me. As the days wore on, I would run into people in the corridor who didn't know what had happened. They too told me how well I looked and asked me had I been away on holiday. This should tell you everything about the culture and conditions that exist for many people working in the NHS. I had started the year with cancer; had undergone an extensive ten-hour operation, local chemotherapy, and a stay in ITU. This was followed up by six months outside and walking on the beach. Yet I looked better than many people who had started the year cancer-free, but spent it working in the department. Also, several people told me that they thought I had been burnt-out. The conditions in which we are working are so dreadful that burnout is ubiquitous; it is assumed that, in the end, it will happen to most of us. It's accepted as something that just comes with the job. Despite the fact that we are trained to deal with physical health conditions, when people began to sense that there was something wrong with me, they didn't even consider a physical health problem.

I returned to my Zumba classes. The first morning I went back I was excited; I told myself that I needed to try not to cry. I left my flat and, as soon as I turned onto the Holloway Road, the tears started. I realised that trying not to cry was not going to happen.

Walking into the changing room at the gym was so familiar it felt surreal. Two women were complaining about how they had put on weight and how they were desperate to lose it. I wanted to tell them that they looked fine. Then I caught sight of myself in the mirror. I couldn't help feeling disappointed with how thick my legs looked. I remembered how skinny they had been immediately after my operation. I could wear anything, and they looked tiny. I had to remind myself that they had thickened with good health and walking, and that now I was going to be able to dance on them.

Upstairs, several people recognised me. I started to cry when I told them where I had been. I tried to explain that I was fine, I was just crying because I was so happy to be back, but I couldn't. They all hugged me.

When Onyeka came upstairs, it was one of those cinematic moments, where she just stopped and stared in astonishment. Then we both hugged each other and cried. I wanted to tell her how happy I was to be there, how I had longed to be back for so long. But I couldn't get the words out.

After the class, she asked me to say a few words. I told everyone how I had been able to sit up after my operation and I felt it was due to the Zumba, that it had helped my fitness, which, in turn, had helped me cope with the operation and the recovery. I said that I wanted to thank Onyeka, but I was glad to have the opportunity to thank all of them: to thank them for all their energy and joy that they had shared with me over the last few years, for I felt that that was one of the things that had got me through my illness. A while later, Onyeka said that it was as if I had been training for what had happened to me. I couldn't help agreeing with her.

In fact, all the things I had done over the previous few years, like all my writing, had helped. They had prepared me, and then sustained me through my illness and recovery. I thought about all my wellness initiatives at work, about my beliefs around the importance of fun and creativity. At times, I had doubted if I was doing any good. I wondered if it had ever really helped anyone. Now, I realised that it had. It had helped me.

After I had been back in London for a few months, I was packing some clothes to go on holiday and came across a pile of black tee shirts, all neatly folded up. They were the ones I had worn all through my illness. My sister had laundered them whilst I was in hospital.

I had a strange feeling when I saw them: a strong, visceral reaction. I decided that I would give them away to a charity shop. I didn't think of them as mine, but as belonging to the jelly belly. With this realisation came another: I had begun to think of the jelly belly as an entity in its own right, some kind of strange creature that had inhabited me for a time. Even more oddly, I didn't think of it as an entirely evil creature. My feelings were much more complex. The jelly belly was more like a trickster that had taken over my body and disrupted my life. He (and, for whatever reason, I thought of it as a he) had forced me to confront my shame and fear, and had then led me down to the underworld.

He may not have taken me on that mythical ferry that crosses the River Styx, but he had left me sitting in the terminal building for a time. And, like a character from a Greek myth, when I returned to the world from the stygian gloom, everything did seem a little brighter and sharper.

I was surprised to discover that, in a funny sort of way, I was grateful to the jelly belly. Also, the writer in me had to admit that he had given me a great story — one hell of a story, actually. Even the doctor in me could not help but acknowledge the beauty and elegance of my medical history. I remembered that when I was a medical student, they would occasionally bring in retired physicians to give us teaching. They would always talk to us about the importance of taking a good medical history. They had learned their medicine in a time far removed from us; a time when they had far less access to investigations.

'Most of what you need is in the history,' they would say. And that was certainly true of me. Looking back, my medical history was perfect. Medicine is an art as much as a science but, in this fast-paced, target-driven world in which we now live, we have neglected that aspect of it.

I thought of the night I had seen my shadow on my bedroom wall, a huge belly and stick-like limbs. I had thought that it hardly looked human. It was easy to imagine that I wasn't looking at myself, but at the shadow of the jelly belly. I wondered why he had chosen me to come and live in. For a moment, I felt almost flattered.

I was proud of the mark that he had left on my body, my long scar and missing belly button. I felt no shame in showing it. Today, showing off your scars is considered an act of bravery; you have earned them after all. But the jelly belly knew, as I showed my scar, what a hypocrite I was. I was a lot more comfortable showing off my scar than I had been showing my abdomen when I thought that I looked fat. Yes, the jelly belly had my measure, both literally and metaphorically.

I may have been grateful to the jelly belly, but I certainly didn't want him to return. So, I thanked him as I put his clothes into a bag, and asked him not to come back again.

A couple of friends told me that, to them, it seemed as if I had been reborn. I understood what they meant. In my wildest imaginings, it sometimes felt that, in some magical way, I had given birth to myself or a new me from the ruptured cyst on my ovary and huge, swollen, pregnant-like belly, with the jelly acting like some kind of fantastical amniotic fluid. As the saying goes, nothing new is ever born without a struggle.

## Afterwards: Hope

When it was all over, people would sometimes ask me if I had learned anything from the experience. People have a need to try and make sense of things, and perhaps there is something in human nature that likes to feel that nothing is ever wasted.

The doctor in me, whilst perhaps not learning something new, had an emotional experience of something that I had known only intellectually before. I had always believed in the importance of good communication and empathy. It wasn't until I was a patient, and a terrified patient, that I understood how vulnerable it is to be in that place and how everything becomes magnified.

I was regularly reduced to tears by small acts of kindness. I cried when the nurse in the day care unit made me a second cup of tea. I loved everyone that looked after me in ITU and the ward. The couple of people who were offhand or brusque left me reeling: distress followed by rage. Nevertheless, I could acknowledge that their behaviour was no different from the way mine had been on any number of occasions when I had been stressed or having a bad day or just preoccupied. But I was surprised how other people's behaviour and attitude affected me so much.

I also thought a lot about how I had managed to deny my symptoms for so long. I had lived in a state of complete cognitive dissonance, and it shocks me still to think how powerful that was, and how I adapted my life to aid my denial.

My attitude towards the medical profession and my own job also changed. I hadn't realised quite how cynical I had become. Over the last few years, I had become increasingly disillusioned. I felt as if I was not doing any real good at all. Instead, I was just stuck in the midst of chaos, failing to achieve anything.

As a patient, I was in awe of all the medical professionals who had cared for me: my GP, gastroenterologist, radiologist, surgeon, anaesthetist and ITU consultant. They had all had their different parts to play. And the sum of those parts was me: still alive and healthy. Whenever I think of any of them, I start to cry with gratitude at the care I received.

I was struck by the job that we all do. I thought of myself and my colleagues, and I remembered the good that we do. We may not be able to deliver the care that we want to, but we are still delivering the best that we can in the circumstances. I had to resist allowing my disillusionment with the system becoming disillusionment with myself or what lay at the heart of the profession. And if, in the end, I leave medicine, I should not regard myself as a failure, but recognise that the current system is failing all of us.

Given that all that I had hoped and prayed for had been granted, something else that changed was my uneasy relationship with hope.

Back in November 2022, when I was very sick but did not know it, I was involved in an initiative with a friend who is a clinical health psychologist, and a theatre company called Wake the Beast. A representative interviewed staff about their experiences and used the material to produce a thirty-minute theatre piece called *In Our Words*. This was performed for an audience of staff and followed by a facilitated discussion. Like Forum Theatre, it involved something I felt passionately about: the use of creativity to explore our experiences of the job. I volunteered to facilitate.

On one of the days, my co-facilitator asked the question, 'What do we need now?' and someone answered, facetiously, 'Hope.'

I thought of growing up as a child in Northern Ireland in the 70s and 80s. It was a time beset by violence, strikes and rioting, but things had changed. They perhaps hadn't been solved, but they had got better. Admittedly, some of them had got worse again — but some had stayed better. Maybe it was important at least to entertain the idea, that things could improve.

I was reminded of hope again while I was at home, recovering. It was a beautiful spring day, and I was out with my sister. I noticed a set of recycle bins that the Salvation Army was using to collect clothing. The slogan written across them was 'Fill Me with Hope.' It made me think about how hope had, unexpectedly, appeared in my life during the four weeks between seeing my GP and my operation: the time that I was talking to Lucy and we both thought that I was going to die, and when the therapist asked me to think of my best-case scenario and then I had found the postcards.

On both those occasions, hope had momentarily sparkled before disappearing. It was complicated, though; perhaps I could argue that my denial of my illness contained false hope in the belief that if only I could diet hard enough everything would go away. What is the difference between hope and false hope, and how do you tell them apart? I thought about this for a long time. Maybe hope is like the stars. You can only really see it when you allow yourself to sit in the darkness.

Before I went back to London, several people told me that I would notice the noise and dirt. I actually didn't. Maybe I had spent so much of my life in noisy places, I could easily block it all out, just as I had always done.

What I did notice, though, that I had never noticed before, was the quiet of the quiet places. I was astonished by quite how quiet some places were. And there are lots of them, even in London, tucked away into the cracks and crevices of the city.

I just have to know where to find them and make sure that I spend a little time there as often as I can.

## Acknowledgements

Thanks to:

My wonderful colleagues: Lucy Parker, Elisha Staun, Duncan Carmichael, Rachel Landau, Sazia Samad, Nora Brennan, Vanessa Georgoulas, Jay Govender, Sid Kona, Natalie Richard, Shabnam Spiers, Firas Abou Auda and Erum Jamall.

All my friends, including Alison Johnston, Vicki Jones, Marc Henry, Sue Gibbons and Karen Hawley.

Onyeka, my wonderful Zumba instructor and friend.

My fantastic writing mentors, Claire Steele and Diane Samuels.

All the professionals who provided care, including Dr Miles Johnston, Dr Dariush Sadigh, Dr Jeevan Kumaradevan, the Peritoneal Malignancy Institute at Basingstoke, including my surgeon, Mr Sanjeev Dayal. And all the other healthcare professionals, including nursing staff, medical staff, healthcare professionals and physiotherapists at the Whittington Hospital, and the Wellington, who took such good care of me.

Constellations Press is a small independent press, committed to publishing works of fiction, memoir and essays. We publish books that boldly reimagine society and celebrate our diverse humanity, adding to the total sum of the world's beauty.

constellationspress.co.uk

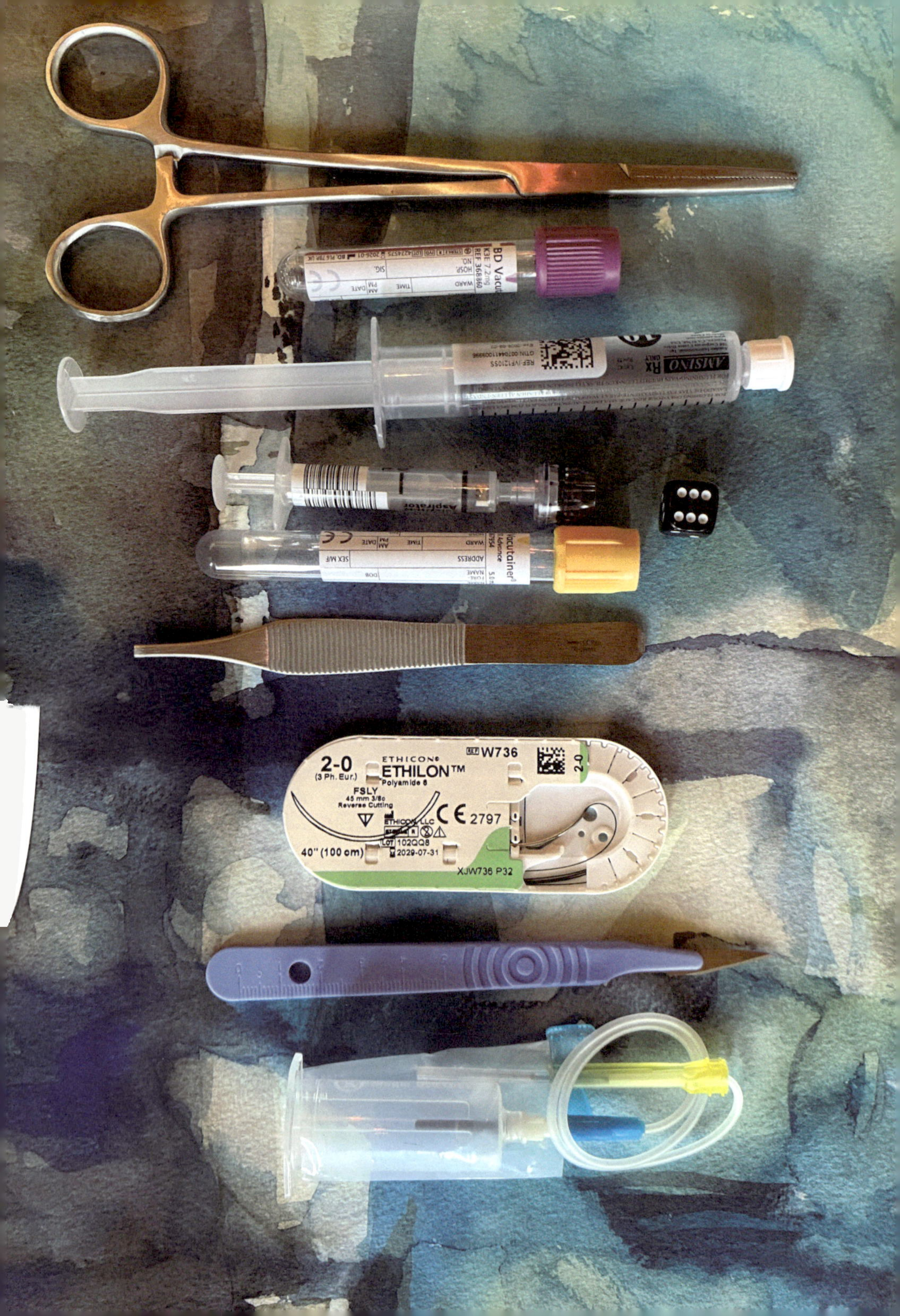
2-0
(3 Ph. Eur.)
ETHICON
ETHILON™
W736
Polyamide 6
FSLY
45 mm 3/8c
Reverse Cutting
2797
40" (100 cm)
102QQ8
2029-07-31
XJW736 P32